Ergonomics Applied to Dental Practice

Juan Carlos Ortiz Hugues, DDS
Certified Ergonomics Assessment Specialist
Private Practice
David, Panama

QUINTESSENCE PUBLISHING

Berlin | Chicago | Tokyo
Barcelona | London | Milan | Mexico City | Paris | Prague | Seoul | Warsaw
Beijing | Istanbul | Sao Paulo | Zagreb

One book, one tree: In support of reforestation worldwide and to address the climate crisis, for every book sold Quintessence Publishing will plant a tree (https://onetreeplanted.org/).

Library of Congress Cataloging-in-Publication Data

Names: Ortiz Hugues, Juan Carlos, author.
Title: Ergonomics applied to dental practice / Juan Carlos Ortiz Hugues.
Description: Batavia, IL : Quintessence Publishing Co, Inc, [2023] | Includes bibliographical references and index. | Summary: "This book teaches dental professionals how to prevent pain and disorders by adopting the four principles of dental ergonomics: knowledge of body biomechanics, using an ergonomic stool, implementing four-handed dentistry, and working with a surgical microscope"-- Provided by publisher.
Identifiers: LCCN 2022017419 (print) | LCCN 2022017420 (ebook) | ISBN 9781647240905 (paperback) | ISBN 9781647240271 (ebook)
Subjects: MESH: Dentistry | Ergonomics
Classification: LCC RK60.7 (print) | LCC RK60.7 (ebook) | NLM WU 100 | DDC 617.6--dc23/eng/20220805
LC record available at https://lccn.loc.gov/2022017419
LC ebook record available at https://lccn.loc.gov/2022017420

A CIP record for this book is available from the British Library.
ISBN: 978-1-64724-090-5

QUINTESSENCE PUBLISHING USA

Quintessence Publishing Co, Inc
411 N Raddant Road
Batavia, IL 60510
www.quintpub.com

5 4 3 2 1

Editors: Marieke Z. Swerski and Leah Huffman
Design: Sue Zubek
Production: Angelina Schmelter

Printed in Croatia

Contents

Preface

Through this text, I hope to broaden your understanding of the science of ergonomics and the impact of its practice in clinical dentistry. In my work as an endodontist, I have experienced the transformative nature of an ergonomic practice. When I first started my clinical practice, I used magnifying loupes for several years before making the switch to the optical microscope. Once I started using the microscope, the change in my posture was almost immediate. This inspired me to learn more about ergonomics and create a practice that was organized, efficient, healthy, and truly oriented to excellence. As I became certified in all levels of both occupational and dental ergonomics, I was able to improve all the details within the office. Not only did I incorporate the microscope, chairs, and other equipment, but I also made substantial changes in the management of clinic staff and patient care. As I acquired and applied this knowledge, I found that pain in my arms and body became reduced and eventually went away.

I began to travel, visiting clinics throughout the United States and Latin America, and saw that ergonomic principles were not being taught in dental school and therefore not applied in practice. Clinicians lacked the knowledge of proper posture, positioning, and organization, and as a result they were setting themselves up for future pain and disorders. The high incidence and prevalence of musculoskeletal disorders in dentistry is no secret, and pain often becomes part of the lifestyle. But it doesn't have to. Understanding the physiology, anatomy, biomechanics, and anthropometric factors that go into designing and organizing an office, as well as the psychosocial and administrative factors, can put you on the right track to address—and even prevent—these disorders. Even better, if these concepts can be applied starting in dental school, dentists can learn correct habits from the start, thereby ensuring a healthy, efficient workflow for the rest of their career.

Ergonomics is a multidisciplinary science that seeks to determine the intellectual, conceptual, and physical changes needed within an office. Throughout this book, you will learn what ergonomics is and why it matters, the most frequent and painful syndromes associated with poor ergonomics, proper postures to prevent these syndromes, and the tools and modifications necessary to build an ergonomic office. The goal is to lay the groundwork for dentists and students to make the changes necessary to prevent musculoskeletal disorders within our profession.

Acknowledgments

I would like to thank all the people who, in one way or another, have contributed to my academic and professional growth throughout my career.

To my parents for sowing the seeds of hard and disciplined work, who through example set me on the path of honesty, perseverance, and a desire to seek education—the most worthy means to grow from the inside out.

To my lovely wife, Susana, who enlivens my life with her love and support.

To my daughter, Mei Helena, who is a fuel in my life to keep working hard with passion.

To all the university professors from my undergraduate degree at the Universidad Latina de Costa Rica, and to all those who trained me as a specialist in endodontics at the Maimónides University of Buenos Aires, Argentina.

To the professionals from all over the world who have guided me with the example of excellence.

To the Academy of Microscope Enhanced Dentistry, which has allowed me to meet brilliant minds, humble and hungry to spread knowledge from the most sincere desire for solidarity and development of other colleagues.

I fell in love with the surgical optical microscope when I first saw it in Dr Santiago Di Natale's office in Buenos Aires, Argentina, in 2006. Finding this precise and excellent technology sparked my passion for the profession. It strengthened my faculties as a clinician; I was able to develop my specialty to its maximum potential, and it makes me perform my work responsibly and with certainty.

To the Palmieri Family, who within the Newton SRL Industria Argentina microscope manufacturer-client relationship found a family. Together we have fed each other ideas, projects, and continuous evolution, based within the framework of a great friendship.

I understand life as an eternal school, where we come to learn and we leave without learning everything, because knowledge is infinite. This book is just a compilation of all my years of study, as well as the study done by many others who were interested in generating knowledge on the beautiful topic of ergonomics. There is a saying: "You can get there faster, but accompanied you can go further."

Introduction

For the dental worker, putting into practice everything mentioned in this text would be a very smart way to improve their quality of life and to succeed in their work. Few texts in the academic area touch on ergonomics and how it directly impacts health and efficiency. The dentist works long hours in awkward and static postures, performing multiple repetitive movements. Their responsibilities are many, and precision is necessary for success.

Knowing what kinds of equipment industries sell and recognizing their shortcomings will go a long way in helping you modify equipment to improve ergonomics. It is essential to recognize the postural and positioning errors that are made daily. This is the only way to correct them and prevent musculoskeletal disorders, which can cause pain and even incapacitate the dentist or dental staff. This entails serious problems—not only physical, but also financial, because pain prevents the dentist from doing a good job, and a day without work is a day without profit in this profession.

It is amazing how simply learning to sit correctly and what positions the human body is designed for can make all the difference. It should be emphasized that the operator's stool is the most important piece of furniture to invest in, because the dentist spends more time in contact with it than with any other element in daily life. Therefore, the stool constitutes the starting point for good ergonomics while working.

Prevention is the best way to guarantee longevity. Therefore, it is crucial to plan time and space for breaks and stretching. Also, the incorporation of the surgical microscope is of utmost importance—there is no other technology that, in a single act, improves the visual capacity and posture of the user. Knowledge of this tool, its settings, and its proper use to enhance ergonomics is extremely important. Training in the use of the microscope in dentistry and its subsequent use in daily practice should be a priority.

The importance of training the assistant should be emphasized as well so the operator can work with their eyes in the microscope and thus eliminate unnecessary movements, increasing productivity and focus on the operative field. Furthermore, it is crucial to consider the assistant's position to prevent them from experiencing the same musculoskeletal pain to which dentists are exposed. They should respect the same prevention laws as the dentist, as these directly influence the efficient workflow that all professionals want in their practice.

With this text, I hope to guide many colleagues to understand why we are a profession with a high risk of musculoskeletal injury. Only with this understanding can we succeed in preventing these disorders and make the necessary corrections that allow for painless and quality work.

General Aspects of Applied Ergonomics

1

Chapter objectives

- Learn the history of ergonomics and concepts of work enhancement
- Understand the importance of ergonomics in work processes within dental practice
- Address ergonomic risks in dentistry
- Address benefits of applied ergonomics within dental practice
- Understand applied body biomechanics in dentistry
- Understand anthropometric factors in the design of equipment used
- Apply ergonomic interventions to avoid musculoskeletal risk factors

Background of Ergonomics

Definitions

There are currently several definitions for this science. According to the Occupational Safety and Health Administration of the United States (OSHA), *ergonomics* can be defined as the study of work. More specifically, it is the science that deals with adapting work to the worker, rather than physically forcing the worker's body to fit the job. It can also be defined as the development and application of a human-system interface that is responsible for the interactions between the human and other elements of a system, such as hardware, software, environment, work, organizational structure, and processes.[1]

Ergonomics and *human factors* are two scientific disciplines that have the common objective of minimizing the risks of injury and disease by optimizing human well-being and creating the holistic conditions for the worker to perform the work efficiently and well. The difference between the two terms is that ergonomics addresses the physical aspect of work and human factors addresses the psychologic aspect.[2]

History

Ergonomics is the integration of a number of diverse scientific disciplines, including physiology, biomechanics, psychology, anthropometry, industrial hygiene, and kinesiology, among others.[3] This science studies musculoskeletal health and its effect on worker performance.[4] With the Industrial Revolution, our society shifted from one based on manual/agricultural production to one based on industry. Accompanying this change was a shift of work from active and dynamic tasks to sedentary tasks thanks to innovations such as machine and computer power.

The momentum of ergonomic advances was due to people such as Bernadino Ramazzini, better known as the father of occupational medicine, who studied medicine with a particular interest in occupational diseases. He was the first to correlate work activities with musculoskeletal disorders. Another contributor to the development of ergonomics as a field was Frederick Taylor, who applied principles of science to improve work efficiency (ie, the scientific study of work). Over the years, countless inventions and concepts have been developed to modernize processes, make them more efficient, and improve the quality of life of the worker.[5]

Since the Industrial Revolution, new ways of working have been imposed in the different societies of the world, accompanied to a great extent by technologic advances that have produced transformation and disruption in the entire labor market. Sedentary work has increased by 83% since 1950, and almost half of the jobs in the United States are currently performed in a sedentary manner.[6]

Applied Dental Ergonomics

Risks in dentistry

More than 70% of dental students complain of musculoskeletal pain in their third year.

Numerous studies have been conducted on the prevalence of pain related to work in dentistry, and the results indicate that more than half of dental professionals experience some form of pain. This pain normally starts as early as dental school (or dental hygiene school), creating bad habits that promote a continuation of the problems throughout one's career. More than 70% of dental students complain of musculoskeletal pain in their third year.[7] Most musculoskeletal disorders are therefore inherited from years of ignorance and lack of training in ergonomics, which is why it is essential to recognize the benefits of an ergonomic dental practice in the early stages of training programs. Bad habits practiced for many years are difficult to eradicate; however, when we learn correctly, we create good habits from the beginning.

In dentistry, it is very common to develop bad posture. Many dentists focus first on the patient's comfort rather than that of the operator or the work team, which is not the best way to avoid work-related risks. Unfortunately, over time, these bad postures can cause some of the most common musculoskeletal disorders. According to the European Agency for Safety and Health at Work, if it is assumed that poor posture in the workplace is the initial factor or symptom developer at the musculoskeletal level, then these disorders are considered *work-related musculoskeletal disorders*.[8]

It is important to use ergonomically designed equipment because this technology can minimize risk factors for developing musculoskeletal disorders.[9] When building a dental office from the ground up, the ideal situation is to achieve harmony between furniture, dental equipment, technologies, space management, safety training, and prevention of musculoskeletal risks. Unfortunately, this is the exception, and many times we start working in places without space design or ergonomic criteria, for which modifications have to be made to achieve some degree of improvement in the ergonomic operation of the office. In this case, we must analyze what is adjustable, what can be redesigned, what must be moved, and what must be purchased or invested in to modify the nonergonomic and transform it to ergonomic.

Benefits of ergonomics

Implementing ergonomics and techniques for prevention of injuries in the field of dentistry can have a profound impact on professionals, including the following[10]:

- Improved management and reduction of musculoskeletal pain
- Prevention of work-related injuries
- Increased productivity
- Reduction of stress at work
- Decreased employee turnover
- Decreased number of sick days
- Safer work environment
- Increased quality of life and job satisfaction
- Increased career longevity

Dental health care workers (dentists, assistants, hygienists) are predisposed to muscle imbalances and the resulting cascade of events. When dentists and their staff are forced to work above their physical limits, a spiral of poor performance begins, and accidents occur more frequently. This results in an increase in operating costs, including the hiring and training of new staff, increased medical costs, and worker's compensation. To avoid the vicious cycle of musculoskeletal disorders, dental professionals must take these risks seriously and take effective action throughout their career.[7] If the dental staff and dentist ignore these consequences due to ignorance or neglect of ergonomic principles, there will be a risk of injury. Ergonomics is designed to minimize worker fatigue and reduce musculoskeletal stress through balanced neutral postures, control of working time movements, and provision and maintenance of healthy work environments. An ergonomic dental practice means an increase in productivity and a decrease of injury risk, which is the main objective of ergonomics.[11]

OSHA proposes standards that can be applied to any occupation and provides basic information on musculoskeletal health and safety; it is a simple guide to understand work standards, which in the same way can be applied to our profession.[7] Because ergonomics is multifactorial, risk factors must be controlled when creating ergonomic intervention programs in any work practice. There are three ergonomic controls as described in Table 1-1. The preferred method to ergonomically control the risk factors is with engineering control because it produces more permanent and efficient results; however, it is also the most expensive method.[12]

Control of work practices, on the other hand, focuses on the way work is developed. In this way, procedures and practices are modified to ensure neutral work positions and safe techniques. To obtain the best possible result, it is necessary to create an ergonomic work protocol in which *(1)* the work environment (what we use to work), *(2)* the task being performed, and *(3)* the focus on the comfort of the operator who performs the work are integrated. This will guarantee an efficient workflow that favors the health of the body parts of the professionals involved (Fig 1-1).

TABLE 1-1 Ergonomic controls

Type of control	General examples	Dental examples
Administrative control	• Equipment maintenance • Job rotation • Rest times	• Organization of agenda • Distribution of procedures • Rest time scheduled with and between patients
Engineering control	• Workstations and work areas • Materials and objects and how these are handled • Office equipment	• Office counter • Surgical microscope • Dental chair delivery system • Ergonomic operator stool • Physical space • Horizontal distances to instruments and tools
Control of work practices	• Focus on the way work is developed • Modification of procedures • Safe working postures • "Ergo breaks"	• Four-handed dentistry • Seated work • Postural education • Transfer of instruments

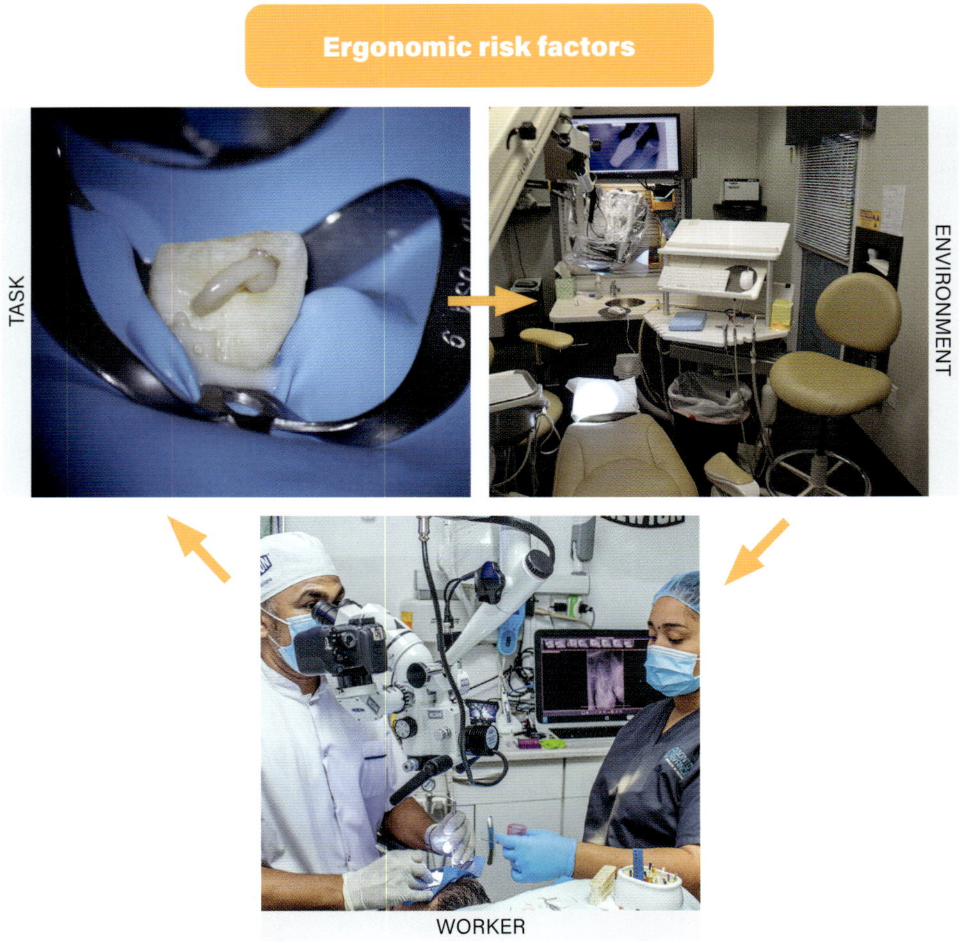

FIG 1-1 Integration of task, worker, and environment.

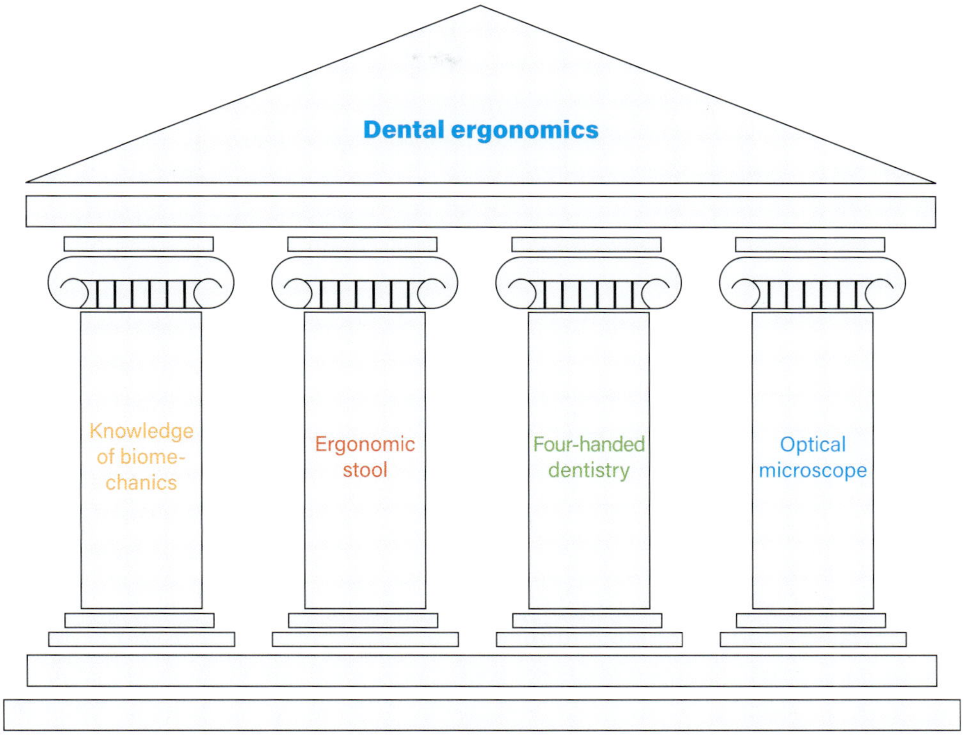

FIG 1-2 The foundations of dental ergonomics include knowledge of biomechanics, an ergonomic stool, four-handed dentistry, and an optical microscope. Without all four pillars, the support is not adequate.

Foundations of dental ergonomics

Much of the information in this book is based on the experience and result of a broad scientific search on how to improve my own dental practice. In the process, I identified four foundations of ergonomics as applied to dental practice:

- Knowledge of body biomechanics
- Ergonomic operator's stool
- Four-handed dentistry
- Surgical optical microscope

The integration of these four foundations within our clinical practice (Fig 1-2) will make our profession one that is productive, simplified, and efficiency-oriented. The key to ergonomic success and the maintenance of healthy systems within our offices is to rely on all four foundations; a deficiency of just one of these prevents the office from being truly ergonomic.

Biomechanics of Posture

Dental work is designed to be carried out in a sitting position, with the dentist remaining sedentary for long working hours. From a biomechanical point of view, this is no different from an office worker; people who work in an office spend approximately 89% of their working time sitting, increasing the risk of developing pathologies such as obesity, high blood pressure, increased cholesterol levels, and heart disease.[13]

In a comprehensive approach to ergonomics, a knowledge of occupational biomechanics is essential to understand the behavior and function of the human body. In this specific case, anthropometrics is a fundamental concept, because dentists often work with equipment, instruments, and technologies that must be selected according to individual anthropometric parameters and physiology. Dentistry is a job with an important physical component, so recognizing the anatomy and physiology of body parts can help us understand the risks of different situations in our profession.

Occupational biomechanics studies the movements and the effects of the forces on objects, applied to living systems within work environments. These forces include gravity, external loads and resistances, and internal forces that act on the skeleton, on the muscles, and in other tissues while performing a job. Ergonomists use their knowledge of biomechanics to understand and improve conditions that may currently be challenging in a work environment.[14]

Personally, when conducting ergonomic assessments and consults in dental offices and dental schools, I refer to the biomechanics of the human body as the missing link within the chain of ergonomics—it is not taught in dentistry. The lack of information and application of clear and simple concepts of ergonomics has a long-term impact on the professional lives of students, and beginning their careers with this knowledge in hand could be very beneficial to their health.

Two of the most important biomechanics concepts in this book are *posture* and *positioning*. It is essential to understand body biomechanics in order to apply ergonomics at work. In a profession such as dentistry in which the worker is seated for long hours in awkward positions (ie, improper posture and positioning), injuries can occur over time.

Mental and bodily fatigue—and of course pain—will restrict the performance of any job.

Biomechanics is taken very seriously in other professions that require mental and physical demand, where performance depends on the state of proper use of the human body. For example, athletes train and stretch methodically with specialized equipment to prevent injury and result in peak performance; dentists should treat their profession in the same way. After all, the goals are the same: to avoid injuries and to perform the work to a high standard in the long term without pain. Mental and bodily fatigue—and of course pain—will restrict the performance of any job.[15]

The discipline of ergonomics teaches us the proper way to use our bodies in dentistry. As we incorporate this knowledge, we will learn to avoid the cycles of poor posture and positioning to which dentists, hygienists, and assistants are subjected. Becoming aware of how the various body parts move, rest, and position themselves during long working hours is a starting point to prevent musculoskeletal disorders and irreversible injuries. In a profession where the worker is seated for long hours, such as dentistry, a proper understanding of the biomechanics of the human body should raise questions such as the following:

- How do I move my different body parts during dental work?
- How many times do I execute and repeat the same movements?
- Am I aware of the neutral sitting posture?
- How am I using my equipment according to my physical parameters?

Asking these simple questions could point to the origin of many of the musculoskeletal pains to which dentists are subjected (which are generally the result of a lack of understanding about how the body really works biomechanically). To result in a healthy long-term outcome, the biology of the body should be respected, and integrated work protocols, technologies, and equipment should be designed for ergonomic purposes.

Kinetics and kinematics

Kinetics and kinematics are two areas of biomechanics that name, evaluate, measure, and study the movement of the components of the body in a state of rest (static) or in movement. Kinetics examines the forces acting on the body during movement as well as the motion with respect to time and forces. These forces include gravity, muscles, friction, and external resistance.

One example of a typical procedure in general dentistry is removing a caries lesion to later place a composite restoration. This procedure may be done using the naked eye or loupes, possibly without an assistant, and may take 1 hour or more depending on the size of the lesion. To perform the procedure, the operator must repeatedly perform multiple motions such as turning the head to the left; tilting to the side, forward, and down to focus on the tooth; moving the upper extremities to reach instruments; rotating the trunk sideways to pick up and put down equipment and tools; and more. At the biomechanical level, the muscles and tendons are working all the time to maintain the neutral posture of the body during the procedure. The motions create internal stress and transmit loads and pressure between adjacent structures within or around a joint at the fulcrum points. The internal forces that are generated in the muscles produce voluntary movements. The efforts and loads necessary to complete the task are transmitted from the muscles to the tendons, ligaments, and bones as well as torque (forces) on the axial axes of rotation in the joints, tension, compression, torsion, or shear within the anatomical structures of the body.[16]

Specifically for the task of caries removal and restoration placement with the naked eye or loupes without an assistant, biomechanically, the internal forces are generated by the musculoskeletal components to keep the operator's head raised and aligned with the spine. Then there are forces (torque) on the axial axes of rotation in the joints or fulcrum points, such as the cervical and lumbar from where the inclination is made to see in the patient's mouth, and the movements from the shoulder joints outward and up to reach. These different inputs, frequently used for this type of activity, do not result in the best use of the operator's body.

The joints and bones behave a certain way when moving the limbs, head, and back according to the axis of movement, axis of rotation in the joint, and the degree of freedom of each joint. Motions create internal stress by *(1)* imposing loads on the involved muscles and tendons in order to maintain the position, *(2)* transmitting loads to underlying nerves and blood vessels, and *(3)* creating pressure between adjacent structures within or around a joint. Dentistry places the operator and staff in working positions with the head forward and down, with movements or esthetic postures that place the joints, muscles, and bones in situations of cyclical fatigue. Positioning like this day after day adds to the potential health issues.

Gravity

Let's address the fundamental force that acts on all body segments all the time: gravity. When they are in direct contact with a surface (eg, in the sitting position), no forces are needed by muscles or ligaments to maintain the position of certain body parts. The surface of the support structure (floor, chair, back, armrest, etc) provides the required equal and opposite "reaction" so that movement does not happen.[17] When there is no support structure, the body must exert force. For example, an endodontist must elevate their elbow over the shoulder at different angulations in the process of shaping root canals in molars. This is a repetitive and sustained posture, and in addition to the internal muscular forces and torque in the shoulder joint, the gravity forces remain, exerting forces on the extremity down and close to the trunk. Similarly with the shoulder, the thrust of gravity on the entire arm is usually passively opposed by the tissues of the joint. This can explain why working with the shoulder elevated or abducted—or even sitting on a stool with no armrest—may increase the possibility of pain and discomfort in the neck, shoulder, and arm.

Statics

Dentistry places the body in prolonged static postures, and this is one of the most dominant risk factors in the profession. *Statics*, a subdivision of kinetics, is the study of bodies when they are at rest and all forces are in equilibrium. The statics of the body are investigated by first reviewing forces, torques, and equilibrium and then applying these conditions to statics in a plane or lever. The principle that governs all static conditions, including static human postures, is that the sum of all forces in any direction (in this case, the vertical—gravity) must be zero. This means that there can be any number of forces acting in the body segment, but these have to sum to zero, with the forces up matching the forces down.

There are several types of forces applied on the body tissues (bones, ligaments, and tendons; Fig 1-3):

- *Compression:* Equal and opposite load directed toward the surface
- *Tension (tensile stress):* Equal and opposite load directed away (outward) from the surface
- *Bending:* Tension and compression applied at opposite sides of a surface
- *Shear:* Load directed parallel to the surface
- *Torsion:* Shear applied along a surface, causing torque

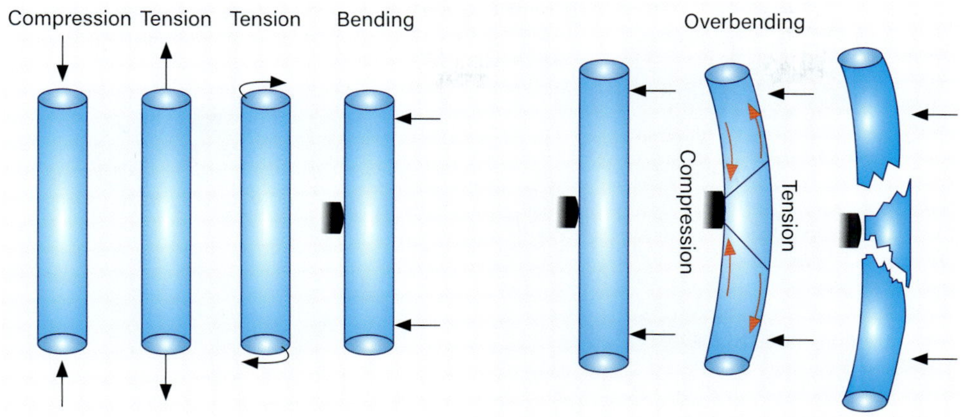

FIG 1-3 Applied forces acting on body tissues.

The way in which these forces are applied externally in static postures will generate an internal force effect on muscles, tendons, ligaments, and joints as a reaction. Examples include shaping a dental canal with the dominant hand, suturing soft tissue, placing layers of composite, preparing a tooth for a veneer, grasping a mirror with the nondominant hand statically prolonged, and tilting the head down to focus on the tooth for minutes or even hours. In addition to these linear support situations, any posture requires an active muscular effort to maintain it. Depending on the posture, the forces can be considerable, and they are regularly accompanied by some unwanted but physiologically unavoidable consequences.

When gravity does not act exactly on the center of a joint, as is generally the case, there is a tendency to rotation (moment or torque) on the axial axis of the joint. The moment and magnitude created in the joint when working will depend on the force and the perpendicular distance from the axial axis of rotation. For example, bending the head forward from the cervical spine is not the same as bending forward from the lumbar spine. The further the line of action of the force of gravity is found from the center of the joint, the greater the moment caused by the gravity. In the case of static posture, when there is no movement, the biomechanical law is applied: The moments that tend to cause rotation on the joint in one direction (clockwise) must be exactly counterbalanced by moments that tend to cause rotation of the joint in the opposite direction (counterclockwise). Leverage is everything. Following the same example, to maintain an upright position when leaning forward from the lumbar spine, torque is counteracted by tension in the back extensor muscles (Fig 1-4). It is easy to understand the nature of musculoskeletal pain in these areas, which will be described in later chapters. To summarize, the effect of postural deviation and the internal forces to sustain the posture combined with the gravitational forces place the different body parts in risk situations. This occurs even if no extra weight is carried on the limbs and is exacerbated when modifying factors (eg, duration, frequency, intensity) are present.

Leverage is everything.

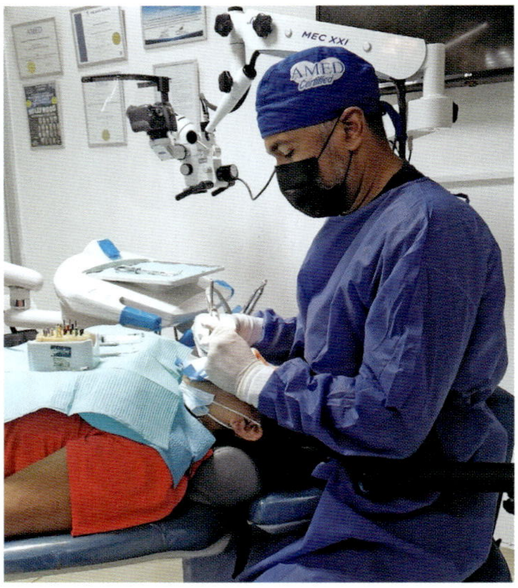

FIG 1-4 *(left)* Applied forces acting on body tissues during naked-eye dentistry include forward head and lower back posture.

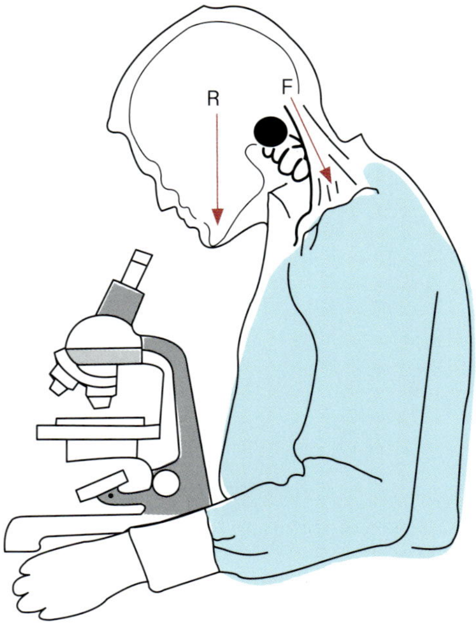

FIG 1-5 *(right)* Static head and neck posture. R = resistance; F = force.

An example of static head and neck posture associated with forward head posture and leverage is when the force of gravity acts in the center of the mass of the head (Fig 1-5). Here, we assume that the axial rotation axis or fulcrum is the atlanto-occipital joint between the head and the first cervical vertebra, the force of control of which is provided by the muscles of the back of the neck. The moment for clockwise rotation is the distance from the thrust line of the muscular force to the axial axis of rotation (lever). In static posture, these two moments must sum to zero. For example, if we estimate that a person's head represents 7% of their body mass, the gravitational force of a 68-kg (150-lb) person is 4.76 kg and, consequently, the force provided for the muscles of the cervical spine should be approximately 9.5 kg. It is important to note that the forces act in the downward direction on the first cervical vertebra.

The compressive strength in the atlantooccipital joint is not just the weight of the head but approximately three times that amount in a forward head posture. In the forward head posture example, if the user leans forward more than 25 degrees, the resistance of the lever increases. As a result, an increase in muscular effort is required, as well as a proportional increase in the compression of the joint. Conversely, if the posture is more erect, the muscle strain and compression in the joint is smaller. The same biomechanical principle applies to the posture of any segment of the body that is not in a relaxed vertical alignment, such as your lower back and shoulder-arm. In this case, we assume that gravity acts on the combined head-arms-trunk in the axis of rotation (L3, L4, and L5). To maintain this static work posture, an equal and opposite force must be provided by the paraspinal muscles of the lower back, in which the lever resistance is many times greater than the force of the lever. This indicates that the lumbar muscles must contract to maintain this posture continuously at a high level, increasing the chances of fatigue, pain, and reduction of blood supply to the region.[18]

The same principles apply to the shoulder. If the task is developed without considering the patient's position in the chair (mouth too far from the operator's hands, patient away from the end of the headrest, or operator in a wrong position), then the operator must keep the shoulders and arms in an elevated position or with the shoulder joint flexed forward or in abduction (laterally) to be able to reach the mouth. To maintain the working posture in the upper limb (upper arm and forearm-hand), an equal and opposite force must be provided by the strength of the muscles that cross the upper part of the shoulder joint (deltoid and brachial biceps). As the arm segments move away from the body, the radius of the gravitational resistance of the lever to the force of the lever is major.[18]

As mentioned previously with respect to the neck and the lower back, from the biomechanical point of view, muscles around the shoulder joint contract more intensely to hold arm positions bent forward or sideways, with the consequential applied forces effects on the compression of the joint, physiologically reducing circulation and blood supply and resulting in general muscle discomfort. As we deviate from the balanced and upright neutral posture, all the body regions exert progressively greater effort to oppose the force of gravity in our body segments.[18]

To achieve a dynamic way of working, it is recommended that dentists move as much as possible during patient treatment to alternate the load; relax the muscles and vertebral column; and promote rests, breaks, and programmed stretching.[19]

The further we deviate from a relaxed posture, the greater effort our bodies must make to oppose the force of gravity.

Applied Anthropometrics

The postures adopted by the dentist and work team are influenced by the design of the workstation.[20] Daily, the dentist uses equipment, tools, and systems—many of which, due to their design features, do not adjust to the operator's body dimensions or the task performed. Sometimes, the dentist may acquire the right tool but use it in the wrong way, something very common due to the lack of understanding of biomechanics, training, and anthropometry guidelines. Applied anthropometrics is responsible for measuring dimensions and other physical characteristics of the human body. The design of the equipment used in dentistry (eg, dental chair, operator's chair, and dental furniture) is obtained from anthropometric data, useful for the following different types of design:

1. Design for extremes
2. Design for adjustable ranges
3. Design for the average
4. Custom design

Design for extremes is used in circumstances where specific design dimensions, such as height and width of a door, are a limiting factor that can restrict the use of places and things for a certain individual. Design for the maximum value of a population should accommodate virtually everyone.

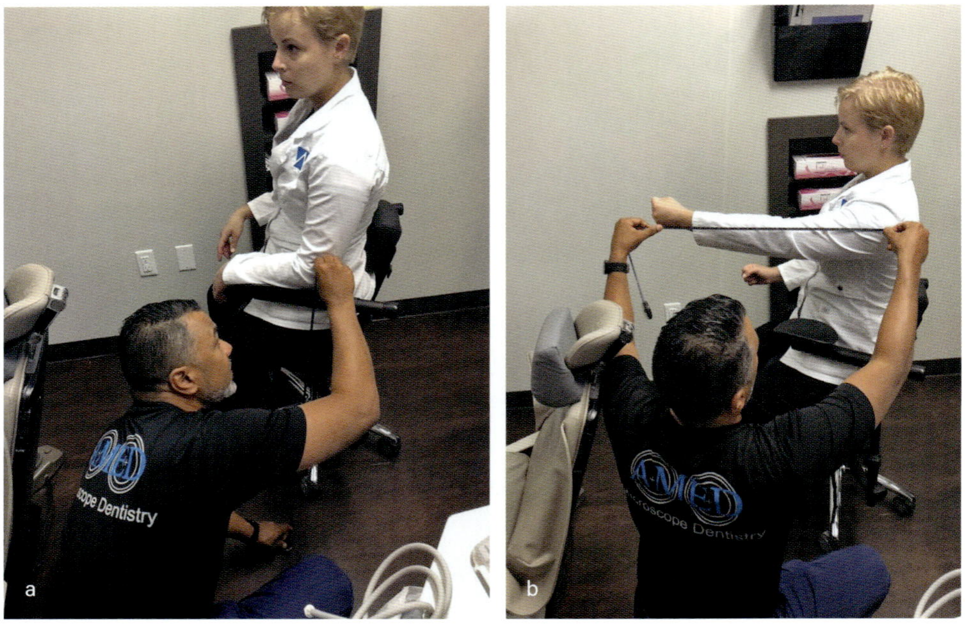

FIG 1-6 Individual anthropometric measurements taken during an ergonomic hands-on session. *(a)* Power zone seated. *(b)* Shoulder to grip.

Designing for an adjustable range refers to certain equipment or workstations that can be adjusted to individuals for their appropriate use. Generally, adjustments are provided that cover a range to accommodate 95% of a 50/50 male/female population, excluding only the smallest 5% of females and the largest 5% of males. Examples include the operator stool and patient chair. This is the ideal design method, but it is not technically or economically viable in all cases.

Designing for the average is a convenient way to group the complex anthropometric variables of the individual. This type of design is used to cover large populations. Male and female percentages of different body segments, weight, distances and other measures are included in preestablished tables and approximate formulas, which can be used to perform the calculations. The objective is that 50% of the female and male population be included in the use of the designed element.[1] Of course custom design is always a possibility to modify or create an item for our own body dimensions or to suit a particular individual or task.

The anthropometric measurements can be applied to give us an idea of vertical and horizontal reaching necessary to avoid wasteful movements that will fatigue the operator and reduce efficiency. During our advanced microscope ergonomics trainings, we provide each participant with a sheet to write down anthropometric data that can then serve as a guide for the most beneficial positions according to their individual measurements. This works for the operator, the assistant, the hygienist, and the office workers. These anthropometric references include the following (Fig 1-6):

- *Elbow to fingertip:* This measurement can help with positioning constant-use equipment and instrumentation for the assistant, hygienist, and operator.
- *Shoulder to grip (middle knuckle):* This measurement can help with positioning frequent-use equipment and instrumentation for the assistant, hygienist, and operator.
- *Power zone seated (elbow to floor):* This can be a guide for the appropriate height of the patient's mouth and head position.
- *Knee height seated:* This is valuable information for the best cylinder height selection for the stool.
- *Distance between elbows and eyes seated:* This indicates neutral head posture in working posture.

As you can see, these sciences provide relevant information to understand the different concepts that will be evaluated throughout this book. Biomechanics explains many of the "whys" of the different musculoskeletal disorders that are experienced regularly among dental professionals. On the other hand, it is useful to understand that the anthropometry applied in the design of the equipment used can help you choose the right equipment or improve existing equipment based on your own body dimensions. For example, when a dental supplier sells an operator stool together with a patient chair and the operator makes the purchase without considering the dimensions, it could result in a mismatch. A tall operator in a chair with a standard cylinder could result in discomfort, and the operator should instead determine if alternative or adjustable equipment is available. The same principles apply to other furniture and spaces in the office.

The work space also should be adjusted in consideration of individual requirements. The working height should be designed to fit the seated working position for the body to achieve a neutral balanced posture.

Another component of effective working design is appropriate placement of instruments. The following are recommended ranges for the horizontal reach of instruments that are constantly or frequently used during seated work to facilitate a healthy and efficient posture[21]:

- *Constant horizontal reach:* 15–17 inches from elbow to fingertip
- *Frequent horizontal reach:* 21.9 inches from shoulder to grip

Organization of workspaces considering the horizontal scope can be a plus when it comes to daily work and the synergy between assistant and operator with respect to the workflow and economy of movements of both. The closer everything we use is, the greater biomechanical advantage to our body parts and work efficiency.

The closer everything we use is, the greater biomechanical advantage to our body parts and work efficiency.

Ergonomic Interventions

The dental workforce is highly susceptible to health issues such as musculoskeletal disorders, which sometimes result in early retirement.[22] It has been suggested that introducing ergonomic interventions can help prevent work-related musculoskeletal disorders by putting all the pieces together. Take a moment to get out of the patient's mouth and analyze your work environment: instruments and tools, how you use them, the office layout and design, administrative management of work time, and training of staff. If we manage our practice to be healthy and efficiently oriented, we may control and prevent this problem, adapting the environment to the dentist and team.[23] The goal of ergonomic interventions is to prevent the development of work-related musculoskeletal disorders by focusing on the worker and factors within the workspace, not the other way around.

The practice of dentistry is highly demanding and challenging due to the amount of manual dexterity, visual acuity, and endurance required to carry out procedures in a narrow, confined, complex, and restricted work area like the oral cavity. It is recommended to follow a systematic approach and step-by-step formula to organize your work at the dental office. Different ergonomic interventions used in other work fields can be applied to prevent risk factors, including phsyical, cognitive, and organizational ergonomic interventions.

Physical ergonomic interventions

Evaluation of working postures

Most of the bad postural habits in dentistry are adopted in dental school, and these vices are carried over into profesional life.[24] These include the way we sit in the operator's stool as well as patient positioning sequences. Because ideal postures are not always adopted by practitioners, clinical ergonomic training and education can be beneficial and reduce the occurrence of musculoskeletal disorders among dentists.[25]

Design factors

Proper ergonomic design and workstation layout can help decrease ergonomic hazards in the job by managing distances, measurments, spaces, temperature, and equipment selection or adjustment in the equipment that we already have. This will both improve productivity at work and reduce work-related musculoskeletal disorders.[26]

Cognitive ergonomic interventions

Psychosocial stress caused by job demands can be managed administratively with appropriate scheduling. This includes not taking on too many patients, organizing time by type of treatment, including scheduled spaces for breaks, and planning time for filling in patient data so the dentist is not rushed or late for break time or time with the next patient. Following a planned and mangageable schedule will reduce work-related musculoskeletal disorders in dental practitioners because psychosomatic stress is also a trigger for some painful syndromes in the musculoskeletal system. Low levels of morale and job satisfaction can contribute as well.[27,28]

Organizational ergonomic interventions

The dentist is not the only member of staff who should be aware of and actively implementing ergonomic principles. The administration, hygienists, and assistants should all receive proper training to promote a healthy work environment. In this way, all components of the work team are organized to establish an orderly, efficient workflow and respect ergonomic laws at all times, which will be conducive to productivity in the office.[29]

Lalumandier et al[30] reported that professionals in all dental specialties show a high occurrence of musculoskeletal disorders, but with variations in frequency and locations. Determining risk factors for work-related musculoskeletal disorders with the support of a group of architects, industrial designers, and ergonomists can help in their prevention. Designing a practice from the point of view of engineering, organization of spaces, and work methodology, starting with body biomechanics, can improve performance and the costs of inactivity due to work disabilities, especially in the areas most affected by the practice of dentistry, such as the head, neck, shoulder, hands, lower back, and wrists.

When I perform dental ergonomic trainings virtually and on site, I begin by observationally verifying all the aspects that form the foundations of dental ergonomics (ie, biomechanics, ergonomic stool, four-handed dentistry, and optical microscope; see Fig 1-2). However, we must always consider the big picture: the job design, the environment, operatory, instruments, and organization. This way, the participant has all the information necessary to maximize the improvement of the workflow, efficiency, and health of the entire team.

We must always consider the big picture.

Assessment of the dentist and workplace should include the following:

- Look for strengths (positive aspects)
- Look for opportunities for improvement
- Present strategies or corrective actions

When looking for the positive factors within the current plane of the evaluation, we seek to reinforce the appropriate working practices and environmental factors that are already being performed well. The core of the evaluation is finding opportunities for improvement. In this way, we can modify the postural and positional aspects of the operator-assistant, correct the use of equipment such as the ergonomic chair or the optical microscope if used, and determine what role the assistant plays and the horizontal reach distances of instruments used constantly and frequently.

The strategies are a set of parameters and corrective recommendations already established to bring the operator-assistant and work team closer to the recommended work method in a simple and systematic way based on evaluations in their work environment. We use images at different angles captured from videos and photographs to help the participant more effectively understand the changes suggested for the ergonomic operation of the office. It is very important to follow up 1 to 3 months after the evaluation to check if there are improvements, using the LEAN method, a well-known work organizational model and cyclical process used in many industries, with the steps of learning, building, and measuring as a form of continuous improvement.[31]

Conclusion

Ergonomics is the study of work and specifically concerns itself with preventing musculoskeletal disorders in workers. These types of disorders are especially prevalent in dentists and dental assistants because of the long hours in prolonged static postures. Preventing pain and disorders must be done by the formation of good and healthy habits and use of properly designed equipment. Implementing the four foundations of dental ergonomics (body biomechanics, an ergonomic stool, four-handed dentistry, and an optical microscope) can help with these goals.

References

1. Hendrick HW. Good Ergonomics is Good Economics. Proceedings of the Human Factors and Ergonomics Society 40th Annual Meeting, 1996; Santa Monica.
2. International Ergonomics Association. What Is Ergonomics? https://iea.cc/what-is-ergonomics/. Accessed 1 March 2022.
3. United States Department of Labor Occupational Safety and Health Administration. Ergonomics: The Study of Work. https://www.oshatrain.org/courses/pdf/OSHAErgonomics.pdf. Accessed 1 March 2022.
4. Pollack-Simon R. All the Right Moves: The Definitive Guide for Integrating Dental Team Ergonomics. Tulsa, OK: Pennwell, 2002.
5. Leirós LI. History of ergonomics, or how the science of work is based on truths taken from psychology [in Spanish]. Rev Hist Psicol 2009;30(4):33–53.
6. Church TS, Thomas DM, Tudor-Locke C, et al. Trends over 5 decades in U.S. occupation-related physical activity and their associations with obesity. PLoS One 2011;6:e19657.
7. European Agency for Safety and Health at Work. OSH in Figures: Work-Related Musculoskeletal Disorders in the EU—Facts and Figures. Bilbao, Spain: EU-OSHA, 2010.
8. Morse T, Bruneau H, Dussetschleger J. Musculoskeletal disorders of the neck and shoulder in the dental professions. Work 2010;35:419–429.
9. Valachi B. Practice Dentistry Pain-Free: Evidence-Based Strategies To Prevent Pain And Extend Your Career. Portland, OR: Posturedontics, 2008.
10. Resnick ML, Zanotti A. Using ergonomics to target productivity improvements. Comput Ind Eng 1997;33(1–2):185–188.
11. United States Department of Labor Occupational Safety and Health Administration. Ergonomics. https://www.osha.gov/ergonomics. Accessed 1 March 2022.
12. Vergara M, Agost MJ. Antropometría aplicada al diseño de producto. Treballs d'informàtica i tecnologia 2015;42. Valencia: Universitat Jaume.
13. Gremaud AL, Carr LJ, Simmering JE, et al. Gamifying accelerometer use increases physical activity levels of sedentary office workers. J Am Heart Assoc 2018;7(13):e007735.
14. Chaffin DB, Andersson GBJ, Martin BJ. Occupational Biomechanics, ed 4. Hoboken, NJ: John Wiley & Sons, 2006.
15. Lindegård A, Larsman P, Hadzibajramovic E, Ahlborg G Jr. The influence of perceived stress and musculoskeletal pain on work performance and work ability in Swedish health care workers. Int Arch Occup Environ Health 2014;87:373–379.
16. Institute of Medicine. Musculoskeletal Disorders and the Workplace: Low Back and Upper Extremities. National Research Council, Institute of Medicine. Washington, DC: National Academy Press, 2001.
17. Chengalur SN, Rodgers SH, Bernard TE. Kodak's Ergonomic Design for People at Work, ed 2. Hoboken, NJ: John Wiley & Sons, 2004.
18. National Research Council and Institute on Medicine (US) Panel on Musculoskeletal Disorders and the Workplace. Musculoskeletal Disorders and the Workplace: Low Back and Upper Extremities. Washington, DC: National Academies Press, 2001.
19. Hokwerda O, Wouters JAJ, de Ruijter RAG, Zijlstra-Shaw S. Ergonomic Requirements for Dental Equipment: Guidelines and Recommendations for Designing, Constructing and Selecting Dental Equipment. Frankfurt, Germany: European Society of Dental Ergonomics, 2006.

20. Todd AI, Bennett AI, Christie CJ. Physical implications of prolonged sitting in a confined posture—A literature review. Ergonomics South Afr 2007;19:7–21.
21. Pheasant S, Haslegrave CM. Bodyspace: Anthropometry, Ergonomics and the Design of Work, ed 3. Boca Raton: Taylor and Francis, 2006.
22. Brown J, Burke FJ, Macdonald EB, et al. Dental practitioners and ill health retirement: Causes, outcomes and re-employment. Br Dent J 2010;209(5):E7.
23. Mulimani P, Hoe VC, Hayes MJ, Idiculla JJ, Abas AB, Karanth L. Ergonomic interventions for preventing musculoskeletal disorders in dental care practitioners. Cochrane Database Syst Rev 2018;10(10):CD011261.
24. Ng A, Hayes MJ, Polster A. Musculoskeletal disorders and working posture among dental and oral health students. Healthcare (Basel) 2016;4:13.
25. Droeze EH, Jonsson H. Evaluation of ergonomic interventions to reduce musculoskeletal disorders of dentists in the Netherlands. Work 2005;25:211–220.
26. Ahearn DJ, Sanders MJ, Turcotte C. Ergonomic design for dental offices. Work 2010;35:495–503.
27. Ylipää V, Arnetz BB, Preber H. Predictors of good general health, well-being, and musculoskeletal disorders in Swedish dental hygienists. Acta Odontol Scand 1999;57:277–282.
28. British Dental Association. Managing stress in dentistry. https://bda.org/stress. Accessed 6 April 2022.
29. Norman R, Wells R. Ergonomic Interventions for Reducing Musculoskeletal Disorders: An Overview, Related Issues and Future Direction. https://www.qp.gov.bc.ca/rcwc/research/norman-wells-interventions.pdf. Accessed 6 April 2022.
30. Lalumandier JA, McPhee SD, Parrott CB, Vendemia M. Musculoskeletal pain: Prevalence, prevention, and differences among dental office personnel. Gen Dent 2001;49:160–166.
31. Brito MF, Ramos AL, Carneiro P, Gonçalves MA. A continuous improvement assessment tool, considering lean, safety and ergonomics. Int J Lean Six Sigma 2020;11:879–902.

The Musculoskeletal System and Cumulative Trauma Disorders

2

Chapter objectives

- **Understand the physiology of the spine and muscles and how they work**
- **Recognize risk factors in dentistry to develop cumulative trauma disorders, such as prolonged static posture, awkward postures, and repetitive movements, among others**
- **Understand the sequence of events to produce a cumulative trauma disorder**

To understand ergonomics, we must review the musculoskeletal system of the human body, because this is the system that will be subjected to cumulative damage when work is not adapted to ergonomic principles. This chapter briefly reviews the anatomy and function of these systems and then describes how these systems are affected by undesirable consequences of nonergonomic positioning.

The Spine

Anatomy

The body is a fascinating machine. The brain, spinal cord, and peripheral nerves regulate all body functions, and together they are the source of the organism's power. The nerves are hypersensitive and reactive to contact, and therefore they must be protected. The skeletal system is the mineralized internal framework consisting of bones, joints, and associated cartilages, and it serves the following functions:

- Serves as the scaffold of the body
- Protects vital organs
- Permits and limits specific movements

The primary purpose of the spinal column is to protect the spinal nerves, and the primary purpose of the skull is to protect the brain. Therefore, the role of the spine is crucial in the maintenance of musculoskeletal health. The spine includes the following elements[1]:

- *Vertebrae:* They are aligned to allow movement with their protective bony wall. In addition, each vertebra is separated by a cylindric disk.
- *Discs:* Hold portions of the vertebrae together and provide shock absorption when the body is standing or sitting.

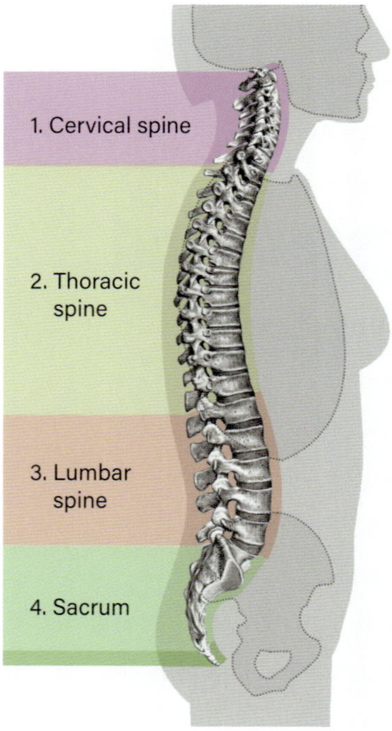

FIG 2-1 Lateral view of normal spinal curvature.

- *Spinal nerves:* Exit through openings between the vertebrae and stimulate the muscles.
- *Ligaments:* Hold the bones together.
- *Muscles:* Help move the bones of the body as they contract and relax.
- *Tendons:* Provide additional anchoring of muscles to the bones.

The spine is composed of a curved stack of 33 vertebrae divided structurally into five regions (with the fused coccygeal vertebrae; Fig 2-1). The disruption of the shape of the spine is a disruption to the nature of the organism, which in the medium or long term can cause a counterproductive effect on the body itself. When observed laterally, the spine looks like an S with concavities and convexities. The cervical and lumbar concavities are called *lordosis*, and the thoracic and sacral convexities are called *kyphosis*. The lordosis and kyphosis are not very mobile, so there should be no major alterations during the normal mobile and static postures in dentistry.

Between each vertebra is a spinal disc (Fig 2-2). These intervertebral discs are fibrocartilaginous cushions serving as the shock-absorbing system of the spine, protecting the vertebrae, brain, and other structures such as nerves. The discs allow some vertebral motion, such as extension and flexion, but they are susceptible to rotational movements.

Intervertebral discs have two components:

1. *Annulus fibrosus:* This is a strong tire-like structure made up of lamellae and concentric sheets of collagen fibers connected to the vertebral end plates. The sheets are oriented at various angles and enclose the nucleus pulposus, holding its position inside.
2. *Nucleus pulposus:* This contains a hydrated gel-like matter, mostly water, that resists compression.

Although both the annulus fibrosus and nucleus pulposus are composed of water, collagen, and proteoglycans, proteoglycan composition improves the capacity of the disc to absorb water. The amount of water in the nucleus varies throughout the day depending on activity. Just as with muscles, the discs require compression and stretching (movement) to be healthy and are susceptible to loads and forces.[2]

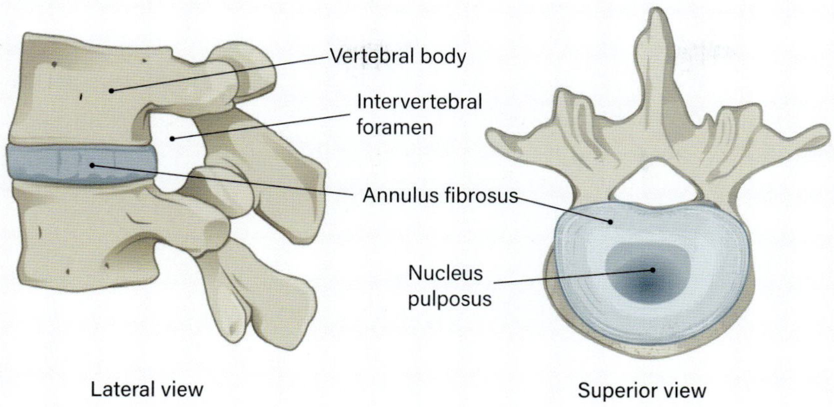

FIG 2-2 Intervertebral discs.

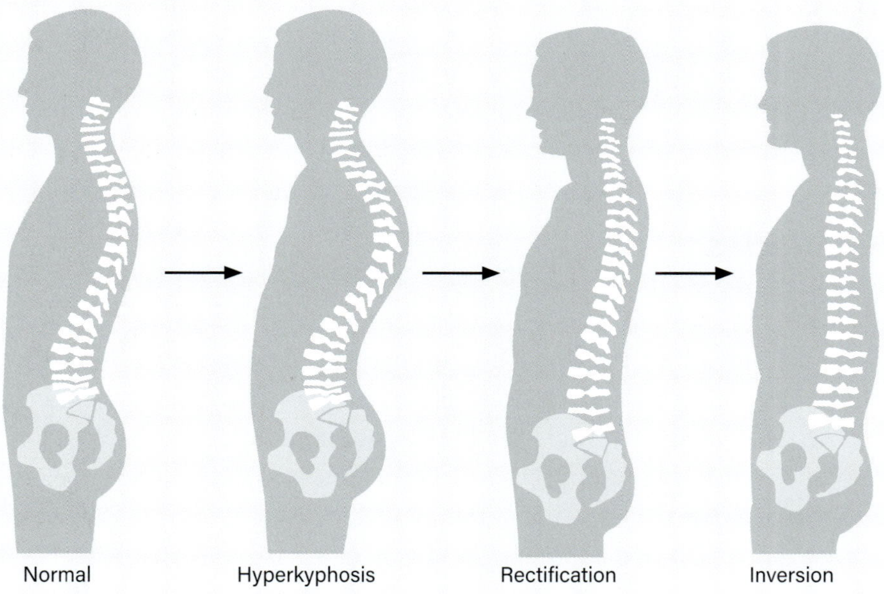

FIG 2-3 Comparison of the normal spinal curvature and other curvatures that can result from poor posture or genetics.

Function

The anatomical nature of the curvature of the spine represents an advantage from a biomechanical point of view and ultimately in maintaining the health of all the structures of the body involved in dental work.[3] However, there are other types of curvatures in the spine that can be generated by poor postures or by genetics, such as hyperlordosis, hyperkyphosis, rectification, and inversion (Fig 2-3). To understand the role of each curve, we must understand its function. The cervical and lumbar lordosis and the thoracic and sacral kyphosis form a counterbalance, which is what allows the top of the body to stay balanced over the center of gravity.

The goal is to maintain the S shape of the natural spine configuration to provide adequate shock absorption. This will reduce stress and tension in vulnerable areas of the back and neck as well as wear and tear and nerve irritation. In dentistry, a suitable operator's stool with a good design and support can help achieve the goal of preserving the natural spinal curve, especially in the lumbar spine, as it provides the support features in sitting postures that balance the spine at its center of gravity by keeping the curvatures neutral.[4]

Dysfunction

Over time, bad posture and positioning at work can develop the so-called tissue memory. Ligaments and other connective tissues that hold the bones together have an elastic property that will expand and contract to its original position. Positions held for a greater amount of time are the ones that sculpt the postures of the body, such as getting a hunched back over time.

The joints and connective tissues are held together by ligaments, which in turn establish a range of limited motion. Ligaments play a key role in stabilizing the bony structures. Movements that exceed that range can produce dislocation, sprains, and pain, which is exacerbated with increased frequency and duration. Conversely, if the joints move less than their optimal range, over time range of motion may become restricted. Therefore, joints should be neither overworked nor underworked.[1]

The Muscles

Anatomy

Muscles are the organs that allow physical work to be performed. Their primary functions include supporting the body, allowing motion, maintaining posture, and protecting internal organs. There are three types of muscle: skeletal muscle, soft muscle, and cardiac muscle. In this book, the focus is on skeletal muscle: the muscle that connects to the bones of the skeleton. A complete muscle consists of many oriented fibers (cells), and each muscle fiber consists of many small myofibers.

Function

Skeletal muscles exert tension when they contract in proportion to their length and maximize their cross-sectional area. There are two types of muscle contractions that are involved in posture and motion: isotonic and isometric. Isotonic contractions involve changing the length of the muscle and are further broken down into eccentric contraction (lengthening) and concentric contraction (shortening). Isometric contractions, on the other hand, do not involve a change in muscle length but are used to maintain a given posture or position. Therefore, they are the most commonly encountered types of contractions in dental work.

Dysfunction

As the muscle stretches, it increases the tension necessary to overcome the elastic resistance of the connective tissue, which surrounds the individual muscles and joins them together. Muscle contraction can be limited by the following factors:

- *When the energy demand exceeds the supply:* The fuel supply to make the muscles work depends on the capacity of the circulatory system.[5] In dentistry, the work-rest-movement cycle can benefit the muscular oxygen supply, the fuel to maintain optimal muscles.
- *When mechanical capacities are exceeded:* The force of muscle output is finite and depends on the number of contractile elements. A task can exceed its mechanical capacity.
- *When the accumulation of waste products alters the muscular function:* This may occur during static muscular activity.

Training to strengthen the muscles can increase the cross-sectional area and the ability to form new muscle fibers to carry out tasks. This is why fitness and core strengthening can be helpful for any physically demanding job, including dentistry.

Repetitive and sustained activity (common in dentistry), fast movements, and movements with a great amount of force can stimulate the muscle receptors. Because skeletal muscle forms 40% of body tissue, it should be no surprise that many of the pains that are experienced daily are of muscular origin. The loss of muscle function that occurs with fatigue increases the risk of musculoskeletal injuries.

Cumulative Trauma Disorders

Risk factors and causes

Stress and fatigue

To understand the impact of stress and fatigue on the body, it is necessary to consider physiology and anatomy. *Stress* and *fatigue* are words used in various ways by ergonomists to refer to temporary states of certain parts of the human body. Stress due to work demands causes fatigue when capacity is exceeded (Fig 2-4). In short, stress is merely the applied load or the demand in the task executed. It can be physiologic or physical and produces fatigue, which results in a decline in physical or mental functions when executing a task.[6]

Fatigue is subjective; it is an unpleasant symptom that incorporates sensations in the whole body, with ranges from fatigue to exhaustion, and it creates a relentless general condition that interferes with the individual's ability to function at a normal capacity.

The crucial point is that stressful work—whether physical or psychologic—generates the same biologic responses; the difference lies in the consequences of stress for mental and physical health and on the reasons why task performance may fail.[7] The terms *stress* and *fatigue* refer to both temporary states of some parts of the body and to chronic states of the person. In both cases, the stress resulting from the

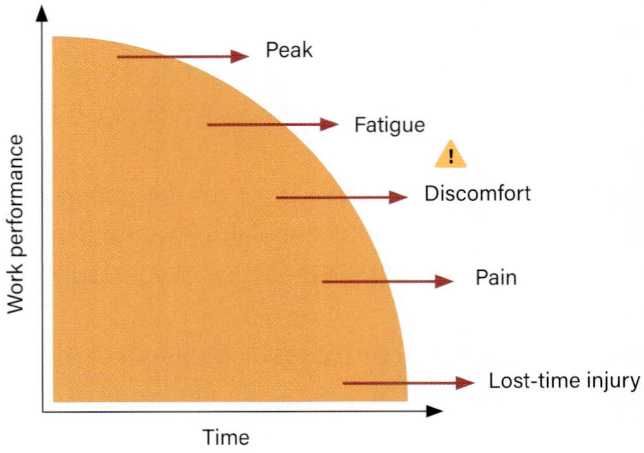

FIG 2-4 Impact of fatigue on work performance. Fatigue is a warning!

execution of a job causes fatigue when the work capacity is exceeded; therefore, stress is the trigger and fatigue is the direct effect due to the physical and mental workload.[7]

Lack of sufficient rest time in dentistry means that damage accumulates faster than the body can repair it.

Sustained microtraumas

Cumulative trauma starts as a microtrauma (ie, a microscopic injury that occurs in certain parts of the musculoskeletal system every day).[8] These damages are in constant repair by our body during rest times. In dentistry, however, rest times are usually insufficient. This can be a result of not scheduling enough time for procedures and factoring in extra time for things such as anesthesia, filing paperwork, and cleaning the operatory; a focus on the volume of patients rather than the quality of care; lack of break times between patients; and many more factors. Insufficient rest time results in damage accumulating faster than the body can repair it. Damaged tissue eventually becomes painful and inflamed, resulting in loss of function.

Risk factors for developing musculoskeletal or cumulative trauma disorders associated with dentistry including the following:

- Long static posture
- Inadequate lighting
- Improper positioning
- Repetitive movements
- Weak postural muscles
- Mental stress
- Awkward postures
- Poor equipment or adjustments
- Poor flexibility

Among these risk factors, pain and dysfunction as a result of static and/or awkward postures cause significant structural damage, especially when there is force, repetition, vibration, or contact/impact stress involved.[9] Microtraumas develop through a series of events and cause a nutrient pathway disorder, which is a primary cause of ergonomic injury.[10]

The human body is designed for movement. Since the Industrial Revolution, when work went from being manual to being sedentary with the incorporation of machinery, the working population has developed numerous musculoskeletal disorders. As a consequence, the United States founded organizations including the Occupational Safety and Health Administration (OSHA) and the National Institute for Occupational Safety and Health (NIOSH) with the objective of developing prevention, intervention, and care programs for these disorders. It is obvious that the way we use our body contributes to this significant increase in work-related pain, especially considering that we live in the computer age, surrounded by smartphones and other devices creating harmful postural habits.

In dentistry, musculoskeletal disorders begin in dental school, with a prevalence among students between 44% and 93% (more common in years 3 and 4 of school than years 1 and 2), and stays with students as they begin their professional careers.[11–13] Studies have suggested that incorporating mandatory ergonomic programs in dental schools at every stage of the theoretical and practical teaching process could be beneficial for the health of students and future professionals. It is not enough to have only a knowledge of ergonomics if these concepts are not practically applied.[14,15] The incorporation of ergonomically oriented teaching could focus not only on the level of execution of the clinical procedure that the student is going to perform but also on postural analysis and the integration of workstations together with ergonomically designed equipment.

Pain and persistent injury

A persistent injury is a very common contributor to chronic pain, though not all cases of chronic pain are the result of a persistent injury. In the purest sense, chronic pain begins as a symptom of an underlying problem, but it then goes on to become THE problem. That is to say, true chronic pain is not a symptom of a condition; it is a condition itself. Pain affects not only the physical function of the worker but also their mental and emotional well-being, which contributes to their overall impairment.[16]

Dentistry is a physically and mentally demanding profession, and a persistent injury may occur sooner or later without prevention. An ergonomic injury is related to pain and dysfunction as a result of risk modifiers. The tissues most often involved are the muscles, nerves, tendons, and/or fascia.

Static and dynamic movement

The musculoskeletal system is subjected to potential functional situations in which it works and adapts in different ways[17]:

- *Dynamic submaximal contraction:* Work cycle that allows replenishment of reserves between contractions.
- *Dynamic maximal contraction:* Work cycle that does NOT allow the required recovery periods, leading to the depletion of reserves and a lower injury threshold.
- *Static contraction:* Work cycle that is sustained with no recovery time; reserves are depleted quickly. This kind of contraction requires proportionally longer recovery periods than dynamic contraction.

A simple example of static muscle work in dentistry is when you hold an instrument. Static work is prevalent in procedures like root canal treatment, periodontal surgery, endodontic surgery, and multiple tooth preparation, which are physically and mentally demanding tasks. Physiologically, this kind of prolonged static task increases pressure inside the muscle, along with the mechanical compression that occludes blood circulation partially or fully. The result is hampered delivery of nutrients and oxygen to the muscles, leading to fatigue and neurologic symptoms over time. It is very different from dynamic work that produces the opposite physiologic result in the body over time. These microtraumas can lead to musculoskeletal disorders such as muscle imbalance, muscular ischemia, trigger points, muscle spasms, and even disc herniation if the situation is not corrected.[8]

OSHA recommends time limits on awkward postures and leverage[18] such as the following:

- Repeatedly raising or working with the hand above the head or the elbow above the shoulder for more than 2 hours per day
- Kneeling or squatting for more than 2 hours total per day
- Working with the back, neck, or wrist bent or twisted for more than 2 hours per day
- Sitting with feet unsupported

If we analyze the parameters of awkward postures suggested by OSHA, we notice how some of them are present in our profession on a regular basis.

On the other hand, dynamic muscle work creates a healthier environment for body repair and health.[19] Dynamic work promotes the removal of lactic acid accumulation and increases pulmonary ventilation, heart rate and blood pressure, blood flow, and oxygen to active muscles while decreasing oxygen to inactive areas. This dynamic movement and blood circulation are necessary to ensure good body physiology. Dental assistants, for example, do more dynamic work when compared with the operator. They spend less working time sitting, stand more frequently, walk, and perform multiple movements in and out of the office.

Even in the most neutral position, muscles maintain static muscle contractions. When the posture deviates from neutral, stabilizing muscle groups of the back and abdomen will be doing extra work to maintain these postures, hence the need to use adequate equipment that provides some type of support to the upper extremities and back during dental work.[20] As the muscles get tired, this prolonged contraction causes muscular ischemia, and this leads to fatigue. When the fatigue is prolonged, it perpetuates a vicious cycle in which the muscles will keep fatiguing, causing cumulative trauma, pain, discomfort, and lost working days, thereby having a direct impact on productivity and performance.[21]

Types of disorders

Muscle imbalance

Human movement is reciprocal in nature: Opposing muscle groups must coordinate for proper movement. Length and strength between opposing muscle groups need to be in balance for normal movement and function. Bad posture is one of the main causes of muscular imbalances, something very common in naked-eye dentistry due to the limitations of the visual information and resolution of the human eye. Naked-eye dentistry encourages the operator to lean forward and down to reach the focal distance of the tooth or oral structure to be worked rather than maintaining a neutral posture.

However, even with the best ergonomic dental magnification equipment, such as a surgical microscope or dental loupes, the operator is frequently placed in bad postures if the biomechanics of the body are not learned properly. Bad posture habits promote the same leaning forward or torso rotations, usually in one direction more than another. This will depend on whether the operator is right- or left-handed, whether they work more at the 9 o'clock or 12 o'clock position, if they use indirect vision with the mirror, and if the patient chair backrest is tilted, among other factors.[22] Over time, muscles can adaptively shorten on one side of the body. This asymmetric posture and the forces caused by this postural imbalance can cause a misalignment of the spine over time, with loss of movement in one direction more than in another. A very common pattern includes shortening and hardening of certain "moving" muscles and weakening of "stabilizing" muscles.[23]

Due to the limitations of the human eye, naked-eye dentistry commonly results in bad posture and is a main cause of muscular imbalance.

Muscle ischemia

Static work increases pressure inside the muscle, and mechanical compression partially or fully occludes blood circulation, so static contraction can decrease blood flow by 60%.[24] This results in hampered delivery of nutrients and oxygen, leading to fatigue or even neurologic damage with time.[25] Muscle pain and fatigue result from the accumulation of lactic acid.

If the range of injured tissue exceeds the repair range due to insufficient rest time, muscle necrosis can result. Because the muscle is injured, the body may use another muscle not designed to do a specific job. This action results in compensatory movement, which can predispose the person to further muscle dysfunctions.[8]

Trigger points

A *trigger point* is a group of muscle fibers found in a constant state of contraction. It feels like a hard nodule and can be painful locally or even cause referred pain at a distant part of the body. In addition, the range of flexibility and movement is decreased in the presence of trigger points. Because trigger points are mainly caused by prolonged muscle contraction, postural asymmetry, and mental stress, they often manifest in both dentists and dental staff.[8]

The affected muscles often display increased fatigability, stiffness, subjective weakness, pain on movement, and restricted range of motion that is unrelated to joint restrictions. As a result, the body initiates a protective muscle contraction or spasm to immobilize the area and prevent a major injury.[26] For this reason, it is common that when faced with chronic pain in the neck, shoulder, arms, wrist, or back, we go to the chiropractor or take analgesic anti-inflammatory drugs to eliminate the pain and return to work. However, these are transitory actions that do not solve the problem (only manage the symptoms, if anything).[27] As shown in Fig 2-5, static posture can lead to many unwanted sequelae.

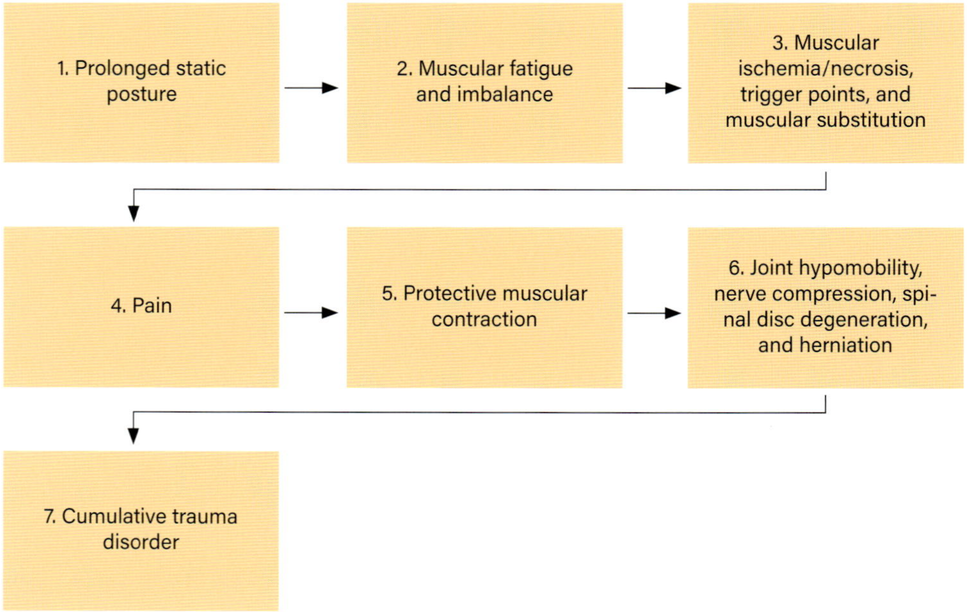

FIG 2-5 Consequences of prolonged static posture.

Prevention

Proper posture

As mentioned throughout this chapter, poor posture is a primary cause of musculoskeletal disorders. Chapter 3 discusses proper posture in depth, and future chapters suggest methods to maintain this posture. The optimal posture of the head is with the ear over the shoulder as seen from the side.[27] Although it is impossible to keep your head in this position when working, unless an optical microscope is used (Fig 2-6), it is important to remember this premise and try to maintain the posture all the time, even if you are not working in the chair. Posture and visual capacity have been shown to deteriorate with age, and maintaining proper neutral head posture becomes more difficult for people with chronic neck pain.[28]

The human body is made for movement.

One of the most complex challenges in dentistry is finding ways to make a mostly static profession dynamic. Because our movements require such stability and precision, the operator gets so focused on the task that they forget to change positions. However, the human body is made for movement, and positions should be shifted whenever possible. It has been suggested that if workload is shifted from one side of the body to the other, it will prevent the obstruction of the nutrient pathway in the muscles.[29,30] Chapter 7 suggests some simple recommendations, including scheduled breaks and stretches, to create a physiologic microenvironment in the body to resolve the static situation in which dentists work.

Taking breaks

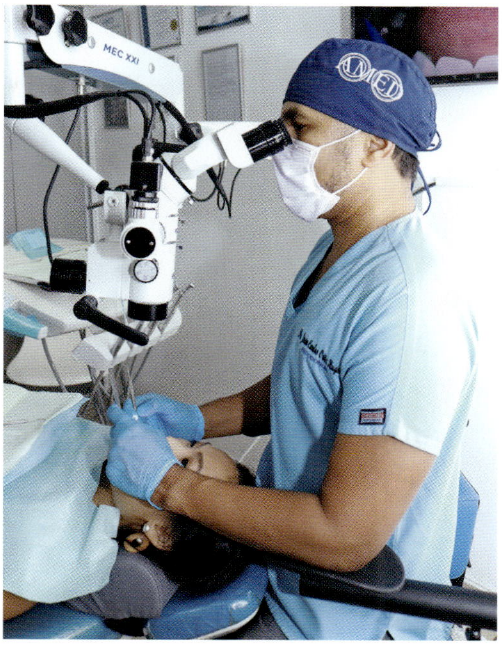

FIG 2-6 Neutral head posture with the use of the optical microscope.

The reality is that dentistry is a very static profession: we work seated for prolonged procedures in the same postures for hours and hours over days, weeks, months, and years. But the good news is that we can find the right tools and prevention methods (eg, rest, ergo breaks, and stretching) to achieve the dynamic impacts our bodies need. By also appropriately managing schedules and rest times, we can minimize the mental and physical fatigue challenges of daily practice.

Generally, any procedure by a general dentist requires working continuously for 30 minutes or more.[31] Fatigue range increases exponentially over time, and recovery range decreases over time. Short and frequent breaks are usually better than infrequent and long breaks because fatigue is minimized and recovery is maximized by cycles of rest and work. The most effective method for tasks that require great effort is to decrease the duration of work periods and provide more rest periods to prevent tiredness. Conversely, a decrease in work intensity is less effective because it will only increase the duration of the work period and provide less time for rest.

Short frequent breaks are better than infrequent long breaks.

However, for low-intensity tasks, it is more effective to reduce the intensity of work to prevent fatigue.[32] The introduction of scheduled rest times during treatment and between patients should be an objective of every dentist. This is how our profession, which is highly demanding physically and mentally, can be efficiently practiced (see chapter 7).

Conclusion

The spine must receive proper support to maintain its curvature, which protects the spinal discs and spinal cord. Frequent poor positioning can disrupt spinal curvature and lead to pain and disorders. In addition, muscles can become fatigued with overuse, reducing function. Cumulative trauma disorders begin small and build up over time; adequate breaks and rest times allow your body to heal and help to prevent stress and fatigue. Ensuring that your body moves dynamically will also help your muscles heal and recover.

References

1. Pollack-Simon R. All the Right Moves: The Definitive Guide for Integrating Dental Team Ergonomics. Tulsa, OK: Pennwell, 2002.
2. Kraemer J, Kolditz D, Gowin R. Water and electrolyte content of human intervertebral discs under variable load. Spine (Phila Pa 1976) 1985;10:69–71.
3. ¿A qué se deben las curvas de la columna vertebral? Medspine: Centro de investigación y tratamiento del dolor de espalda. https://www.medspine.es/curvas-columna/. Accessed 3 March 2021.
4. De Bruyne MA, Van Renterghem B, Baird A, Palmans T, Danneels L, Dolphens M. Influence of different stool types on muscle activity and lumbar posture among dentists during a simulated dental screening task. Appl Ergon 2016;56:220–226.
5. Huang MJ, Nosaka K, Wang HS, et al. Damage protective effects conferred by low-intensity eccentric contractions on arm, leg and trunk muscles. Eur J Appl Physiol 2019;119:1055–1064.
6. Puriene A, Janulyte V, Musteikyte M, Bendinskaite R. General health of dentists. Literature review. Stomatologija 2007;9:10–20.
7. Bridger RS. Introduction to Ergonomics, ed 2. London: Taylor & Francis, 2003.
8. Valachi B. Practice Dentistry Pain-Free: Evidence-Based Strategies to Prevent Pain and Extend Your Career. Portland, OR: Posturedontics, 2008.
9. Pîrvu C, Pătraşcu I, Pîrvu D, Ionescu C. The dentist's operating posture: Ergonomic aspects. J Med Life 2014;7:177–182.
10. EU-OSHA. OSH Wiki. Musculoskeletal disorders and prolonged static sitting. https://oshwiki.eu/wiki/Musculoskeletal_disorders_and_prolonged_static_sitting. Accessed 3 March 2022.
11. Thornton LJ, Barr AE, Stuart-Buttle C, et al. Perceived musculoskeletal symptoms among dental students in the clinic work environment. Ergonomics 2008;51:573–586.
12. Pope M. Muybridge lecture. In: Proceedings of the International Society of Biomechanics XIVth Congress. Paris, France: International Society of Biomechanics; 1993. p. 10–3.
13. Diaz-Caballero AJ, Gómez-Palencia IP, Díaz-Cárdenas S. Ergonomic factors that cause the presence of pain muscle in students of dentistry. Med Oral Patol Oral Cir Bucal 2010;15:e906–e911.
14. Thornton LJ, Stuart-Buttle C, Wyszynski TC, Wilson ER. Physical and psychosocial stress exposures in US dental schools: The need for expanded ergonomics training. Appl Ergon 2004;35:153–157.
15. Sasso Garcia PP, de Araujo Gottardello AC, Presoto CD, Bonini Campos JA. Ergonomic work posture in undergraduate dentistry students: Correlation between theory and practice. J Educ Ethics Dent 2015;5:47–50.
16. Foster NE, Thomas E, Bishop A, Dunn KM, Main CJ. Distinctiveness of psychological obstacles to recovery in low back pain patients in primary care. Pain 2010;148:398–406.
17. Habibzadeh N. Physiology of distinct modes of muscular contraction. Int Physiol J 2018;1(3):1–8.
18. United States Occupational Health and Safety Administration. Ergonomics for Trainers. https://www.osha.gov/sites/default/files/2018-11/fy12_sh-23543-12_ErgoforTrainers-TTTProgram.pdf. Accessed 3 March 2022.
19. Kroemer KHE, Grandjean E. Fitting the Task to the Human, ed 5. Philadelphia: Taylor & Francis, 1997.
20. Valachi B, Valachi K. Mechanisms leading to musculoskeletal disorders in dentistry. J Am Dent Assoc 2003;134:1344–1350.
21. Cailliet R. Soft Tissue Pain and Disability, ed 3. Philadelphia: F. A. Davis, 1996.
22. Kihara T. Dental care works and work-related complaints of dentists. Kurume Med J 1995;42:251–257.
23. Chaitow L, DeLany J. Clinical Application of Neuromuscular Techniques, Vol 1: The Upper Body, ed 2. London: Churchill Livingstone, 2008:35–40.
24. McNeil CJ, Allen MD, Olympico E, Shoemaker JK, Rice CL. Blood flow and muscle oxygenation during low, moderate, and maximal sustained isometric contractions. Am J Physiol Regul Integr Comp Physiol 2015;309:R475–R481.
25. Encyclopaedia of Occupational Health & Safety. Muscular Work. https://www.iloencyclopaedia.org/component/k2/item/487-muscular-work. Accessed 3 March 2021.
26. Donnelly JM, Fernández-de-las-Peñas C, Finnegan M, Freeman JL. Travell, Simons & Simons' Myofascial Pain and Dysfunction: The Trigger Point Manual, ed 3. Philadelphia: Wolters Kulwer, 2019.
27. Saunders D, Saunders RL, Kraus SL, Woerman A. Evaluation, Treatment, and Prevention of Musculoskeletal Disorders. Philadelphia: Saunders Group, 1995.
28. Falla D, Jull G, Russell T, Vicenzino B, Hodges P. Effect of neck exercise on sitting posture in patients with chronic neck pain. Phys Ther 2007;87:408–417.
29. Lehto TU, Helenius HY, Alaranta HT. Musculoskeletal symptoms of dentists assessed by a multidisciplinary approach. Community Dent Oral Epidemiol 1991;19:38–44.
30. Finsen L, Christensen H, Bakke M. Musculoskeletal disorders among dentists and variation in dental work. Appl Ergon 1998;29:119–125.
31. Chaikumarn M. Working conditions and dentists' attitude towards proprioceptive derivation. Int J Occup Saf Ergon 2004;10:137–146.
32. Gael S. Job Analysis Handbook for Business, Industry and Government. New York: Wiley, 1988.

Sitting Posture

3

Chapter objectives

- **Learn the appropriate sitting posture according to biomechanical principles**
- **Understand the consequences and disorders that can result from sitting with incorrect posture for prolonged periods and how to prevent them**
- **Learn what kinds of tools are available to help adopt an ergonomic sitting posture**

Posture is one of the most important ergonomic risk factors. In an occupation like dentistry, the head is usually in a slight forward posture, even when using magnification devices like loupes. Over time, the suboccipital muscles can adaptively shorten to keep the head in this bad posture, which means excessive work for the stabilizing and moving muscles of the spine.[1,2] This chapter discusses proper and improper sitting posture in dentistry and the problems that may result from prolonged static posture.

Neutral Sitting Posture

Description

According to the 2012 National Health and Nutrition Examination Surveys, 70% of people spend 6 or more hours each day sitting down.[3] Because seated work represents a risk factor for musculoskeletal disorders, it is essential to learn the correct forms of sitting and the ideal equipment for it; this should be taught as early as dental school so correct posture can be adopted from the beginning of one's career. Numerous epidemiologic studies have shown that people who work in sitting positions have a greater chance of suffering from back problems. When comparing standing work positions versus sitting work, the big difference lies in the pressure of the intervertebral discs, due to the loss of the lumbar protective curve. It is essential to prevent flattening of the lumbar curve in the lower back[4] (Fig 3-1).

To understand proper posture, we must also understand that spinal curves are interdependent; therefore, a change in one curve will result in a change to the curves above and below it. To maintain a healthy neutral posture during seated work, we must respect the nature of our machine—the human body. As reviewed in chapter 2, the spine is S-shaped with definitive curves, lordosis and kyphosis, which must be respected. The cervical C6 and C7 and lumbar L4 and L5 are the most critical areas of the spine, because they are the ones that function as fulcrum points. These sections have

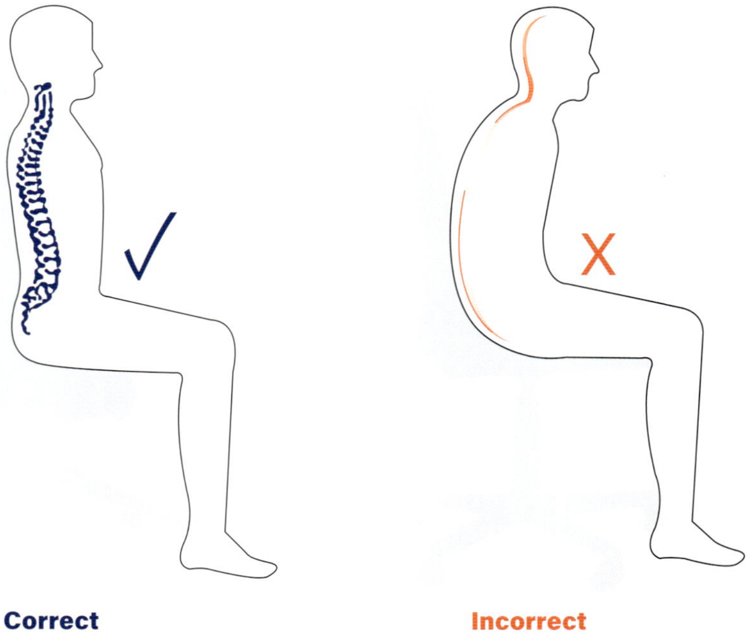

FIG 3-1 Correct and incorrect sitting posture.

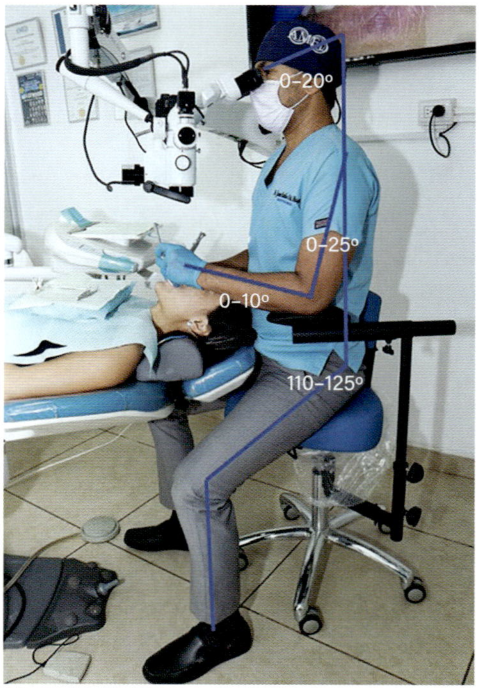

FIG 3-2 Neutral sitting posture. The pelvis should be positioned with an angle of 110 to 125 degrees to the knees. The pelvis rotates forward, maintaining the lumbar curve and releasing the discs.

greater mobility, and they are the ones that present the highest incidence of pain among dentists. This is because the forward and rotational movements necessary to observe the oral cavity during naked-eye dental treatment are carried out from these areas.[5] Rotational force and load in dentistry are aggravated by a sustained slouching posture, which flattens the spinal curves. These postures are becoming more recognized as risk factors for musculoskeletal disorders.[6]

Due to anthropometric differences, the ideal sitting posture will vary slightly between operators; however, it is important to define a successful ergonomic starting point[7] (Fig 3-2). To achieve a normal (neutral) sitting posture, there should be a slight curvature in the lower back, shoulders above the hips, elbows relaxed at the sides, and forearms approximately parallel to the floor. The neutral position of the head is ears over the shoulders.[7] However, this position can be difficult to achieve unless an operative optical microscope is used (Fig 3-3).

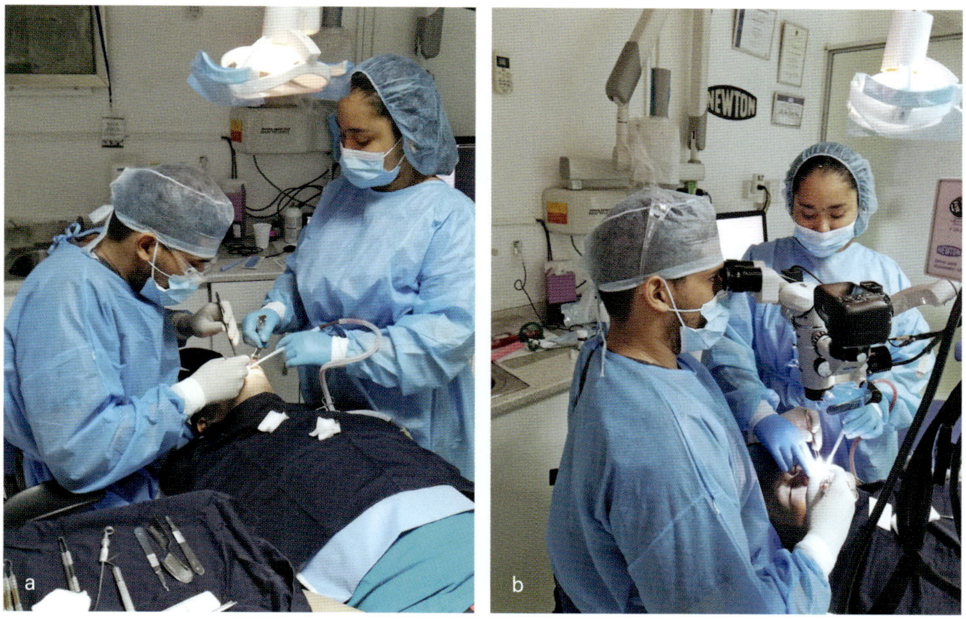

FIG 3-3 *(a)* Posture without microscope. *(b)* Posture with microscope.

Dr Bethany Valachi, a pioneer in ergonomics applied to dentistry, has described the recommended postural working ranges in a very precise and science-based way.[8,9] When using magnification, the operator should obtain postures of the head no more than 20 degrees forward, with a maximum of 25 degrees (see Fig 3-2). The angle of the hips should be greater than 90 degrees to decrease pressure on internal organs and maintain the lumbar lordosis.[10] Recommended hip angles range between 105 and 125 degrees, depending on the operator stool used and whether the chair tilts. The thighs should bend slightly down, with feet firmly planted on the floor and aligned with the orientation of the knees (see Fig 3-2). It is considered acceptable to reach forward from the shoulders with the arms a maximum of 25 degrees and abduction of the arms at 20 degrees.[8] The forearms must be parallel to the floor or lean slightly up to 10 degrees, which will allow greater torque production of the elbow and facilitate better posture.

As an endodontic specialist who immersed himself in clinical practice without a surgical optical microscope for the first 5 years of my career, I can say that the postural changes achieved when I incorporated the microscope were immediate. They were also improved by incorporating the ergonomic chair and perfected by studying the basics of advanced occupational ergonomics.

Neutral posture of upper extremities

Neutral shoulder posture is often defined as elbows to the sides, relaxed shoulders, and forearms parallel or nearly parallel to the floor. This position is difficult to maintain in dentistry, but there is a safe range of shoulder work. The upper arm can abduct outward and sideways no more than 20 degrees and with a forward range of 25 degrees maximum.[8] It is important that the occlusal surface is at the elbow level or within 4 cm above it.[8]

Arm abduction or shoulder elevation will typically occur when the patient is at a higher level than this position, especially when working at the 9 o'clock to 10 o'clock positions. To control the adequate neutral posture of the shoulders and arms, it is essential to consider both the armrests of the dental stool and the position of the patient in the dental chair. Choose a stool with adjustable armrests, and utilize a position that allows for the elbows to be relaxed on both sides. If the armrest is higher, the arms will be pushed up from the shoulder, generating fatigue in this zone. An important parameter to know is the height of the patient in the dental chair. The patient's mouth should be at the level of the operator's hands or slightly higher, in the area of power of the operator or hygienist.

Tools to achieve neutral posture

Maintaining a neutral posture of the lower back is essential in the prevention of pain in the area and to preserve a long professional practice. The most important thing is to maintain and respect the spinal curves when sitting. In dentistry, the best way to help maintain the neutral position of the pelvis—and consequently the head—is to use an ergonomic stool with the appropriate characteristics, as well as a surgical optical microscope[11–13] (see Fig 3-3). The magnification offered by the microscope allows for correction of the most problematic postural situations in dentistry.

The human body has its postural limitations, so an appropriate ergonomic chair or stool can play a major role in maintaining the health of the pelvis and supporting the postural muscles of the back. Think of each part of the body as a tool with a specific function. For example, a fork would not be used to cut a piece of raw meat; in the same way, it is not recommended that the back structures assume positions for which they are not designed. This is why it is crucial to select the right stool that puts the pelvis in its most neutral position to balance the spine, reduce muscle tension, and decrease pressure on the intervertebral discs.[14] Remember, we spend more time sitting on the dental stool than we do sleeping in our beds. The selection and purchase of a dental stool should include serious consideration of its comfort and, above all, the support it provides to the anatomical structures.

We spend more time sitting in the dental chair than we do sleeping in our beds. Invest in a dental stool accordingly.

The ergonomic stool facilitates maintenance of the natural curve of the lower back by providing a slightly forward inclination,[15] placing the hips higher than the knees to allow the pelvis to rotate forward to a more neutral position (like when standing). This position promotes a healthy environment for the lower back during the working day.[16] The use of an ergonomic stool is key to reaching the health and productivity we desire in our practice; it is an investment worth every penny. All the features to look for in a good ergonomic stool are described in detail in chapter 6.

The evidence suggests that back pain in the workplace can be prevented by ergonomically designing the tasks. Some specific ergonomic risk factors that should be prioritized in a redesign include the following[17]:

- Repetitively loading weight
- Loading objects from the floor in rotating positions
- Jobs with high physical demand
- Prolonged sitting posture at work (> 95% of the workday)
- Nonneutral trunk positions sustained for > 10% of the cycle of work in repetitive jobs

Injury risk in the workplace is mostly due to work habits (80%) rather than work design (20%). However, both are key to managing injuries. Therefore, the way we do dentistry—the knowledge and habits adopted while performing work—are most important, but the design of the office, schedules, organization, and tools we use also influence our ability to build a stress-free practice.

Active versus passive sitting

The body responds to sedentary work with two types of sitting postures (see Fig 3-1): passive and active. *Passive sitting* is the classic sitting posture of slumping and sliding the bottom forward in the chair; it expends little energy, so it is less tiring. The big danger, though, is that the load is put on the spinal discs.[4,9] The spinal curve becomes flattened, significantly increasing the load on the back muscles.[9,18] It can also stretch and permanently elongate the iliolumbar ligaments, which decreases the stability of the spine.[19] Over time, these ligaments, muscles, and soft tissues can stretch and shorten to fit the stooped work posture, keeping the spine in this unbalanced posture. Muscle fatigue and degeneration of lumbar discs or hernias are consequences of this position in the long term.[20]

An *active* type of sitting produces the opposite result in the body. However, it expends considerable energy and therefore cannot be maintained for a long time unless the muscles are trained to do so by a strong core. No disc loading apparently occurs, so pain when sitting for long periods is less probable. The proper function of postural muscles such as the erector spinae muscles and the transverse abdominal muscles (those running horizontally around the midsection, similar to a corset) can play a big role in sustaining this sitting posture, but there will eventually be a feeling of tiredness due to the exhaustion of energy sources, and the individual will automatically revert to passive sitting.[4]

Poor Sitting Posture

Description

Prolonged awkward postures are one of the main risk factors for musculoskeletal disorders in dentistry.[21,22] The microdamage of the muscular and vertebral discs over time depends on frequency and duration of this poor posture: The more time spent in this bad posture, the greater the risk of painful musculoskeletal disorders. Physiologically, this classic static contraction present in dentistry may result in a switch to anaerobic metabolism, which increases the acid formation that then decreases efficiency of energy mechanisms. Ultimately, this will result in the peripheral fatigue and failure to sustain a contraction, as well as mental fatigue due to monotony, difficulty of the task, and workload.[23]

Prolonged awkward postures are one of the main risk factors for musculoskeletal disorders in dentistry.

In a prolonged static posture of the muscles that extends the spine (see chapter 2), the discs are compressed, and intradiscal pressure is increased. This pressure is exacerbated when the conventional flat seats of industrial dental stools are used, which don't promote the opening of the hip angles.[24] When this happens, nutrition pathway obstruction in the discs occurs, and a painful syndrome in the lower back develops over time. This means that there is an interrelationship between the biomechanics of the human body and the equipment we use in dentistry.

Leaning forward

Prolonged static postures result in counteracting torque or rotational force, especially when tilting the head forward. Torque or rotational force occurs when a system goes into imbalance. The main perpetrator of this torque generation is the head, which usually weighs from 11 to 14 pounds. The weight of the head and its position have significant influence on body movements. In dentistry, in an effort to achieve direct oral cavity visualization, operators tend to lean forward. In a normal situation in naked-eye dentistry and with loupes, forward head posture exceeds 20 degrees. There may also be side bending and neck twisting during prolonged working situations, often causing mild or moderate muscle pain in the neck or lower back. Poor posture at work may or may not be recognized immediately as the source of this pain. In fact, this postural change may go unnoticed until fatigue results due to sustained microtrauma over time.[25]

There are two types of forward tilt by the operator when performing diagnosis and dental treatment. The first is described as head tilt with fulcrum positioned in the cervical neck area (ie, bending the neck to lean forward). Torque due to tilting of the head forward is predominantly resisted by the erector spinae muscle, which originates in the sacrum and is inserted in the posterior occipital notch of the skull. The second type of forward tilting produces a greater impact. It is common to observe operators lean forward from the pelvis even more than 30 degrees to achieve a line of vision more favorable to the oral cavity. In this position, the torque is increased so that 2.5 m/kg, which must be resisted by the lumbar region.

Risk factors

The challenges in dentistry that result in poor posture include not following a systematic positioning sequence, not using a proper stool, not using the microscope, and working without an assistant. All of these actions/inactions can impact the musculoskeletal system, joints, and intervertebral discs with time.

As a trainer and specialist in ergonomic assessments, I have found serious basic deficiencies in the way of sitting for assistants, hygienists, and dentists. Many of these are related to basic rules as simple as sitting at the correct end of the chair or seat or leaning on the backrest, not to mention the use of arm supports. Even if a stool has proper armrests, they may go unused because the operator is not accustomed to using them or is unaware of their benefits. Part of the problem is that operator stools that come along with dental chairs may have a poor design with deep, flat seats and backs without lumbar support.

The further from the spine the workload is, the more torque that will be required by the body to maintain the position. This translates to greater musculoskeletal and spinal disc fatigue, a common pattern when the head of the patient is positioned far away from the operator's hands. Leverage is everything in ergonomics, so greater tension will be produced in the muscles of the trunk and spinal discs.[26] A very important action to prevent tension and back pain is working closer to the patient.[7,9] This could be a challenge when horizontal reach distances are not respected, work is performed without a dental assistant, the office furniture is organized poorly, or when equipment is ergonomically inappropriate. An ergonomic stool with a tilting mechanism or a saddle stool could be very useful in these circumstances to help the dentist get closer to the patient's mouth by giving enough space for the legs to fit under the chair headrest.[27]

Problems Caused by Poor Sitting Posture

A correct posture is necessary to prevent imbalances in other parts of the body.[9] In fact, the spine and hips, to some extent, affect the movements of the torso and head. The posture of the trunk should be analyzed in terms of average orientation and alignment of spinal and pelvic segments. A prolonged sitting posture tends to transfer the load to the spinal discs, placing the operator at a higher risk of disc damage than in standing jobs.[7] This is why the challenge of maintaining balanced spinal curves is greater in sitting work positions.

The prolonged static posture entails muscle group contractions (erector spinae in the lumbar and cervical) required to maintain the common positions of the operator, which can decrease blood flow in and out of the area due to compression. This results in muscle degeneration of bone and nerve tissue in the affected area.

Herniated discs

One of the most frequent postures when performing naked-eye dentistry is the leaning forward posture to see the working area. When this happens, the nucleus of the spinal discs pushes toward the rear wall of the discs. If the chronic micro-trauma in awkward sitting postures continues and pain is ignored and not treated, the problem could easily get worse, even to the point of needing surgery to relieve pressure on the nerve. This results in missed working days, diminished productivity, and disability of the dental staff.[28]

A herniated disc (also called a bulged, slipped, or ruptured disc) can be one of the severe consequences of awkward postures in dentistry. Herniated discs can occur in any part of the spine; they occur as a mechanical displacement of the nucleus out of the annulus, pressing the spinal nerves and producing pain and movement restriction (Fig 3-4). Herniated discs are more common in the lower back (lumbar spine) but also occur in the neck (cervical spine). Prolonged static postures, such as forward head posture, will predispose one to herniated discs.[29]

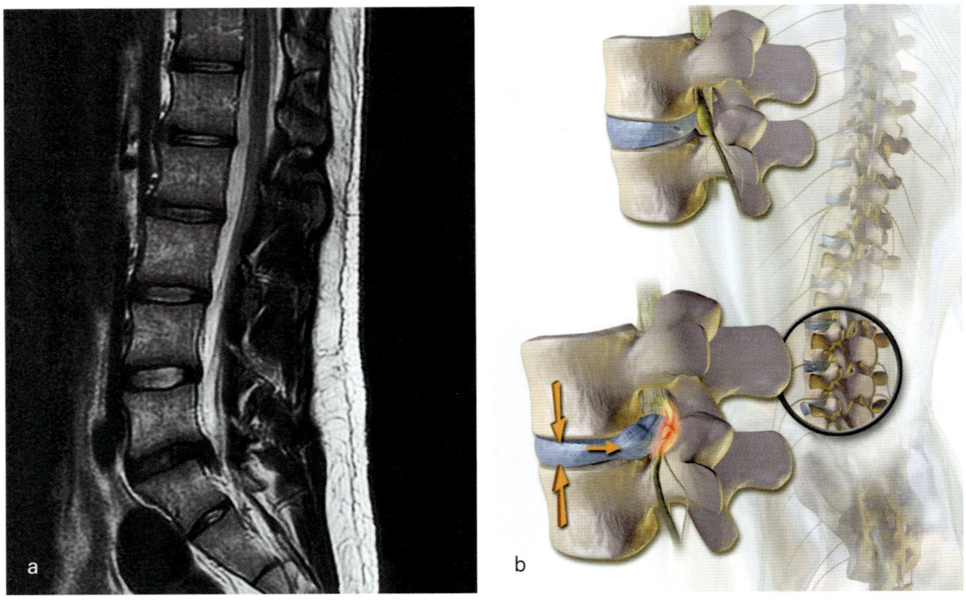

FIG 3-4 *(a)* Radiograph of a herniated disc. *(b)* Illustration of a herniated disc. Note how the hernia presses against the spinal cord, causing nerve compression and pain.

Mechanical stress placed on the spine is higher in sitting positions than in standing ones.[30] When we are sitting with no lumbar support, as often happens in dentistry, the pressure on the discs increases dramatically. Some studies show that dentists and hygienists tend to lean forward at least 30 degrees for more than half of the work hours.[31] Incidentally, the load on the lumbar discs always decreases when the back is in contact with the lumbar support, reinforcing the relevance of a good selection of an ergonomic stool for the operator and assistant.[8]

For a true disc herniation to occur, the trunk must be inclined frequently and in a repetitive fashion; usually the lumbar L3, L4, and L5 are the most damaged vertebral discs.[32] Dentists and hygienists spend more than half of their working time in this kind of forward position leaning from the lumbar spine,[31] and this posture can be an etiologic mechanism of a herniated disc.[33]

Older people often get a herniated disc as a natural part of the aging process. It can also happen as a repetitive motion injury.[34] A neutral posture is the only way to prevent this outcome. Another factor to consider in this profession is that discs require movement to stay healthy, so prolonged static muscle contractions should be minimized. This can be accomplished with an adequate sitting position and physical exercise as well as adequate rest, stretching, and programmed exercises built into the administrative working controls (see chapter 1). The idea is to make this static profession more dynamic, and this can be achieved with programed breaks to walk, breathe, move, and stretch.

Lower back pain

Every year, between 10% and 17% of adults in the United States experience lower back pain; however, within dentists and hygienists, the prevalence of this ailment is 37% to 63%.[9] Lower back pain is a primary cause of occupational disability, and it costs the economy $90 billion annually.[9]

Back pain is not a disease, but it can be a symptom. It can be the natural response of a tissue to biomechanical loads, which can disappear quickly after several episodes, or it can be a symptom of a weakening, degenerative condition that leads to a long-term disability. *Acute back pain* can last a few weeks and is usually a response to biomechanical loads or their consequences, such as muscle fatigue. It can also be a consequence of herniated vertebral discs, tearing of muscle fibers, or ligament tension. *Subacute back pain* can last up to 3 months and is indicative of a new injury or relapse or that something more complex is happening. *Chronic back pain* lasts more than 3 months and can be part of an even more complex disorder. In this instance, the initial injury causes tissue damage, which changes the mechanical function of one or more segments and leads to a cascade of maladaptations, in which each problem causes another problem. In these cases, specialized services may be required in rehabilitation.

To avoid back pain, it is necessary to reduce excess stresses and strains on the back and ensure that the back is strong and supple. Clearly, there is not much that ergonomics alone can do to decrease the burden of back pain or disability in society; however, the incidence of the ergonomic risk factors for certain lower back pain and some of these risk factors can be modified to reduce the exposure of people who suffer from it.

The sitting position, one of the best studied occupational postures, is considered to be a strong risk factor for lower back pain. In the 1960s, Alf Nachemson published extensively on pressure conditions in the human intervertebral disc. Using in vivo measurements, he showed that the total load on the disc increases by about 38% in the seated as compared with the standing position in young adults.[35] The extensor muscles and stabilizing muscles play a key role in prolonged static postures because they can become fatigued or weakened. The abdominal transverse muscle, the abdominal oblique muscle, the quadratus lumborum muscle, and other key muscles play a very important role in lower back stabilization and maintenance of the lumbar curve.[9,15,32]

The main sources of pain come from the spinal discs, capsule joints, posterior ligaments, and back muscles. Another source may be nerve compression. There is also some evidence that those suffering from chronic back pain exhibit an inefficient contraction of the transverse abdominal muscles, muscles that play a very important role in the stiffness of the trunk during postural movements.[33] The soft tissues of the spine are exposed to heavy loads and, over time, this drifts in a cascade of maladaptations that cause problem after problem. Vascular damage due to disc degeneration causes nerve root damage, which results in a syndrome of chronic pain.[36]

There is also a direct relationship between back pain and muscle fatigue: Those with back pain suffer from muscle fatigue more frequently than those without back pain. Pain occurs directly as a result of receptor stimulation of pain in the muscles because of biomechanical changes that accompany fatigue, and indirectly by an increase in soft tissue load in the lumbar spine. Those who suffer from chronic lower back pain are at a higher risk when faced with tasks that involve repetitive loads, carrying weights from the front of the body, leaning the trunk forward, or working with the trunk extended; all of these require sustained activity of the back extensor muscles.[37]

Muscle fatigue and musculoskeletal disorders

Musculoskeletal disorders are the most frequent occupational health-related problems that are still prevalent in current dental practice, despite changes in equipment and surgery design.[38] In dentistry, shoulder girdle stabilizing muscles—especially the middle and lower trapezius muscles—tend to fatigue quickly with forward head, rounded upper back, and elevated arm postures. The direct consequence is that other muscle groups (upper trapezius, levator scapula, and upper rhomboids) start overworking to compensate for the fatigue of the stabilizing muscles.[39] This explains the classic "tension neck syndrome" among dentists as a result of the muscular imbalance,[40] which is explained in more detail in chapter 4. Adaptive shortening of the lower back muscles is a consequence of leaning and bending for a long time and can lead to muscle imbalance. This inappropriate posture is the primary cause of bulging disc or hernia.[8,9]

According to a broad questionnaire of 450 German dentists from varying specialties, the prevalence of musculoskeletal disorders ranged from 65% to 92%. The most affected body regions included the neck, shoulders, and lower back. This was significantly higher than the general population, and studies in other countries have found similar restuls.[41–43] In the United States, about 30% of all dentists who retire early are forced to do so due to musculoskeletal disorders.[35] In a study performed by the University of Glasgow, 189 dentists retired due to injury or illness. The average retirement age in this group was 51 years, with a range from 31 to 62 years. The main injury was musculoskeletal disorders (55%), followed by behavioral disorders (28%).[44]

In the United States, about 30% of all dentists who retire early are forced to do so due to musculoskeletal disorders.

Conclusion

Maintaining proper posture is crucial to preventing musculoskeletal disorders. As in all professions where the worker spends most of the day seated, you must have proper lumbar support to maintain the spinal curves. The most important tool at your disposal is a properly designed stool (see chapter 6). In neutral posture, the shoulders should remain above the hips, the ears above the shoulders, the elbows relaxed, and the forearms parallel to the floor. Avoid leaning forward from the back or the neck and twisting/rotating from the trunk. The seat of the stool should be angled down to keep the knees below the hips. If improper posture is maintained over time, it can result in herniated discs, lower back pain, muscle fatigue, and more.

References

1. Pollack-Simon R. All the Right Moves: The Definitive Guide for Integrating Dental Team Ergonomics. Tulsa, OK: Pennwell, 2002.
2. Leirós LI. History of ergonomics, or how the science of work is based on truths taken from psychology [in Spanish]. Rev Hist Psicol 2009;30(4):33–53.
3. Owen N, Healy GN, Matthews CE, Dunstan DW. Too much sitting: The population health science of sedentary behavior. Exerc Sport Sci Rev 2010;38:105–113.
4. Mandal AC, Haaksma E. Homo Sendens: The seated man and back complaints. The Hague: Product development The Hague Clinic, Back Training & Advisory Centre. Laboratory Back Quality Europe.
5. Gaowgzeh RA, Chevidikunnan MF, Al Saif A, El-Gendy S, Karrouf G, Al Senany S. Prevalence of and risk factors for low back pain among dentists. J Phys Ther Sci 2015;27:2803–2806.
6. Kwon Y, Kim JW, Heo JH, Jeon HM, Choi EB, Eom GM. The effect of sitting posture on the loads at cervico-thoracic and lumbosacral joints. Technol Health Care. 2018;26(suppl 1):409–418.
7. Karwowski W, Marras WS. The Occupational Ergonomics Handbook. Boca Raton: CRC, 1999.
8. Chaffin DB, Andersson GBJ, Martin BJ. Occupational Biomechanics, ed 4. Hoboken, NJ: John Wiley & Sons, 2006.
9. Valachi B. Practice Dentistry Pain-Free: Evidence-Based Strategies to Prevent Pain and Extend Your Career. Portland, OR: Posturedontics, 2008.
10. Rucker LM, Sunell S. Ergonomic risk factors associated with clinical dentistry. J Calif Dent Assoc 2002;30:139–148.
11. De Bruyne MA, Van Renterghem B, Baird A, Palmans T, Danneels L, Dolphens M. Influence of different stool types on muscle activity and lumbar posture among dentists during a simulated dental screening task. Appl Ergon 2016;56:220–226.
12. Harvard Heath Publishing. Why Good Posture Matters. https://www.health.harvard.edu/staying-healthy/why-good-posture-matters. Accessed 10 March 2022.
13. Comes C, Valceanu AS, Rusu D, et al. A Study on the ergonomical working modalities using the dental operating microscope (DOM). Part II: Ergonomic design elements of the operating microscopes. Timisoara Medical J 2010;60:97–102.
14. Neumann DA. Kinesiology of the Musculoskeletal System: Foundations for Physical Rehabilitation. St Louis: Mosby, 2002.
15. Hokwerda O, Wouters JAJ, de Ruijter RAG, Zijlstra-Shaw S. Ergonomic Requirements for Dental Equipment: Guidelines and Recommendations for Designing, Constructing and Selecting Dental Equipment. Frankfurt, Germany: European Society of Dental Ergonomics, 2006.
16. Hedman TP, Fernie GR. Mechanical response of the lumbar spine to seated postural loads. Spine (Phila Pa 1976) 1997;22:734–743.
17. Waddell G, Burton AK. Occupational health guidelines for the management of low back pain at work: Evidence review. Occup Med (Lond) 2001;51:124–135.
18. Harrison DD, Harrison SO, Croft AC, Harrison DE, Troyanovich SJ. Sitting biomechanics part I: Review of the literature. J Manipulative Physiol Ther 1999;22:594–609.
19. Kumar S (ed). Biomechanics in Ergonomics. Philadelphia: Taylor & Francis, 1999.
20. Valachi B, Valachi K. Mechanisms leading to musculoskeletal disorders in dentistry. J Am Dent Assoc 2003;134:1344–1350.
21. Chaitow L, DeLany J. Clinical Application of Neuromuscular Techniques, Vol 1: The Upper Body, ed 2. London: Churchill Livingstone, 2008:64–66.
22. Cailliet R. Neck and Arm Pain, ed 3. Philadelphia: F. A. Davis, 1991.
23. Krueger GP. Sustained work, fatigue, sleep loss and performance: A review of the issues. Work Stress 1989;3:129–141.
24. Ortengren R, Andersson GB, Nachemson AL. Studies of relationships between lumbar disc pressure, myoelectric back muscle activity, and intra-abdominal (intragastric) pressure. Spine (Phila Pa 1976) 1981;6:98–103.
25. Augustson TE, Morken T. Musculoskeletal problems among dental health personnel. A survey of the public dental health services in Hordaland [in Norwegian]. Tidsskr Nor Laegeforen 1996;116:2776–2780.
26. Bogduk N. Clinical anatomy of the lumbar spine and sacrum, ed 3. Sydney: Churchill Livingstone, 1999.
27. Valachi B. Operator Stools: How Selection and Adjustment Impact Your Health. Dentistry Today. https://www.dentistrytoday.com/operator-stools-how-selection-and-adjustment-impact-your-health/. Accessed 10 March 2022.
28. Cleveland Clinic. Herniated Disk (Slipped, Ruptured or Bulging Disk). https://my.clevelandclinic.org/health/diseases/12768-herniated-disk. Accessed 10 March 2022.
29. Huang CC, Kuo PJ, Hsu CC, et al. Risk for cervical herniated intervertebral disc in dentists: a nationwide population-based study. BMC Musculoskelet Disord 2019;20:189.
30. Alamin TF, Agarwal V, Zagel A, Qeli A. The effect of standing vs. variants of the seated position on lumbar intersegmental angulation and spacing: A radiographic study of 20 asymptomatic subjects. J Spine Surg 2018;4:509–515.

31. Marklin RW, Cherney K. Working postures of dentists and dental hygienists. J Calif Dent Assoc 2005;33:133–136.
32. McGill S. Low Back Disorders: Evidence-Based Prevention and Rehabilitation. Champaign: Human Kinetics, 2002.
33. Hernia discal. Saludalia. https://www.saludalia.com/pruebas-diagnosticas/hernia-discal. Accessed 10 March 2022.
34. Fardon DF, Milette PC; Combined Task Forces of the North American Spine Society, American Society of Spine Radiology, and American Society of Neuroradiology. Nomenclature and classification of lumbar disc pathology. Recommendations of the Combined task Forces of the North American Spine Society, American Society of Spine Radiology, and American Society of Neuroradiology. Spine (Phila Pa 1976) 2001;26:E93–E113.
35. Nachemson A, Elfström G. Intravital dynamic pressure measurements in lumbar discs. A study of common movements, maneuvers and exercises. Scand J Rehabil Med Suppl 1970;1:1–40.
36. Bridger RS. Introduction to Ergonomics, ed 2. London: Taylor & Francis, 2003.
37. Gilad I, Kirschenbaum A. About the risks of back pain and work environment. Int J Ind Ergon 1986;1:65–74
38. Moodley R, Naidoo S, Wyk JV. The prevalence of occupational health-related problems in dentistry: A review of the literature. J Occup Health 2018;60:111–125.
39. Novak CB, Mackinnon SE. Repetitive use and static postures: A source of nerve compression and pain. J Hand Ther 1997;10:151–159.
40. Levangie PK, Norkin CC. Joint Structure & Function: A Comprehensive Analysis. Philadelphia: F. A. Davis, 2005.
41. Ohlendorf D, Naser A, Haas Y, et al. Prevalence of musculoskeletal disorders among dentists and dental students in Germany. Int J Environ Res Public Health 2020;17(23):8740.
42. Lin TH, Liu YC, Hsieh TY, Hsiao FY, Lai YC, Chang CS. Prevalence of and risk factors for musculoskeletal complaints among Taiwanese dentists. J Dent Sci 2012;7:65–71.
43. Khan RS, Ahmad F, Merchant MS. Prevalence of work related musculoskeletal disorders (MSD) among dentists. Int J Contemp Med Res 2017;4:1208–1211.
44. Brown J, Burke FJ, Macdonald EB, et al. Dental practitioners and ill health retirement: Causes, outcomes and re-employment. Br Dent J 2010;209:E7.

Pain Syndromes in the Upper Limb

4

Chapter objectives

- **Recognize the muscle imbalances to which dentists are subjected**
- **Understand how job positions, ergonomic equipment adjustments, and exercises can positively or negatively affect musculoskeletal health of the upper extremities**
- **Understand the biomechanics of the upper extremities and the risk factors associated with them**

Bad posture, inappropriate movements, and imbalances in the neck and shoulder can result in the three most prevalent painful syndromes in dentistry:

1. Tension neck syndrome
2. Rotator cuff impingement
3. Trapezius myalgia

In addition, there are several cumulative trauma disorders of the upper limb that dentists may be afflicted by.

The neck and the shoulders should move properly during daily work activities; it is essential for the dental professional to promote healthy movements and postures to protect this sensitive area of the body. The neck and shoulder are closely related and mutually influenced by the musculoskeletal system and the neuromuscular system. Therefore, it is very difficult to study syndromes of the neck without considering posture and shoulder movements. Neck pain and shoulder pain among US dentists have a prevalence of 73% and 65%, respectively.[1]

Neck and shoulder syndromes are largely related to day-to-day activities such as the following:

- Constant lifting of shoulders to move the dental chair lamp when working with the naked eye
- Nonsystematic positioning by the operator, assistant, and hygienist
- Abduction of arms (moving the arms away from the midline more than 20 degrees) to reach instruments and equipment of frequent or constant use
- Working without a dental assistant (to collaborate and hand instruments to the dentist)
- Lack of organization within the office
- Overscheduling patients and lack of rest

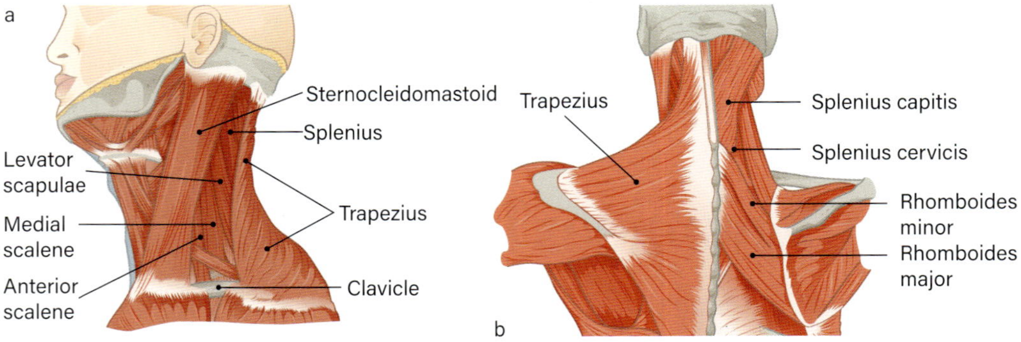

FIG 4-1 *(a and b)* Muscles of the neck and upper back.

To maintain optimal neck and shoulder musculoskeletal health, it is essential to understand how various work postures, positions, ergonomic equipment adjustments, and exercises can affect musculoskeletal health positively or negatively. When the head is freely positioned on top of the vertebral spine, the downward pressure is released into the body. As a result of this posture, an elongation and broadening of the torso are generated. Eliminating this pressure greatly reduces back pain, breathing problems, and neck pain.[2] Prevention of these painful syndromes can be accomplished in the following ways:

- Understanding biomechanics in dental work
- Properly using ergonomic devices in the office, such as an ergonomic stool and optical microscope
- Maintaining body symmetry when working
- Respecting horizontal reach distances

Tension Neck Syndrome

Muscle tension in the neck is a common situation in dentistry. The neck contains flexible muscles that support the weight of your head (Fig 4-1). These muscles can be injured and irritated from overuse. Neck pain can also sometimes be attributed to worn joints or compressed nerves, but tension neck syndrome typically refers to muscle spasms or soft tissue injuries. The top of the spine is also located in the neck and can be a source of pain.

Neck tension can come on suddenly or slowly. Ongoing neck tension that comes and goes over the course of many months may have less noticeable causes. Inflammation of the neck muscles ensues due to overload and an unstable neck posture.[3]

Dental work exposes the operator to a range of postures and movements that can affect the muscles in the neck. Biomechanically, tilting and holding the head in specific positions leads to muscle overuse that can cause these problems. Because the visual capacity of the human eye has limitations, it is impossible to focus on teeth in an upright position with more than 25 to 30 cm of focal distance. As a result, the dentist or hygienist commonly leans toward the mouth, causing this poor posture. This problem can be mitigated with the proper use of a microscope, which should be taught in dental school to promote a better posture (see Fig 3-3).

Symptoms

The symptoms of neck tension include the following:

- Muscle tightness
- Muscle spasms
- Muscle stiffness
- Difficulty turning your head in certain directions
- Pain that worsens in certain positions

Forward head posture is one of the contributing factors to tension neck syndrome and most of the ergonomics issues in dentistry (see chapter 3). This position is common due to years of poor posture, such as holding the neck and head in an unbalanced position forward to gain better visualization during treatment (see Fig 3-3). In fact, neck pain is associated with any job where the head is positioned forward 20 degrees or more for 70% of the working time.[2] On average, a dentist works with the head forward at least 30 degrees for 85% of working time in the office.[4] For this reason, it is worth cultivating a regular awareness and knowledge of the neutral position of the head (ears on shoulders at side view) when working. This means the operator must have more positional awareness. Having a dental assistant can also help in this regard.

Forward head posture is one of the contributing factors to tension neck syndrome and most of the ergonomics issues in dentistry.

Over time, forward head posture can lead to muscle imbalances as the body tries to adapt and find efficient ways to hold the head up for straight-ahead vision. Some muscles become elongated and weakened, whereas other muscles become shorter and tighter. The *Spine-Health* article "Workplace Ergonomics and Neck Pain" by Gavin Morrison[5] provides a very helpful explanation of how the muscles work and become affected by this posture.

Muscles that elongate and weaken

Common muscles that elongate and weaken due to long-term forward head posture include the following:

- *Deep cervical flexors:* These muscles lengthen as the chin tilts away from the neck.
- *Erector spinae (lower cervical and upper thoracic):* When these muscles lengthen and lose strength, they are less capable of keeping the neck and upper back from hunching forward.
- *Shoulder blade retractors:* Weakened trapezius and rhomboid muscles force the shoulder blades to tilt forward, further contributing to hunched shoulders and forward head posture.

Muscles that shorten and tighten

Muscles that commonly shorten and tighten due to long-term forward head posture include the following:

- *Suboccipital muscles:* These four muscle pairs help with head rotation and extension. They continually contract to keep the head tilted up and looking straight ahead during forward head posture.
- *Chest muscles:* As the muscles in the upper back become elongated as the shoulders round forward, the chest muscles may become shortened and tight.
- *Levator scapulae muscles:* If the shoulder blade starts to tilt forward and rotate up with rounded shoulders, the levator scapulae muscles may become shortened.

This explains the importance of maintaining an adequate posture in the head and neck and why, biomechanically, we must think about incorporating habits and technologies that promote proper posture. All of these muscle groups work overtime in prolonged forward head posture. Additionally, the monotonous tasks, intense concentration, and high level of pressure in daily work frequently also result in a psychosocial reaction.[6]

Rotator Cuff Impingement

Symptoms and diagnosis

Symptoms of shoulder/rotator cuff impingement include pain in the shoulder when performing certain movements such as reaching, lifting objects and working above the head, or separating the arm from the midline of the body. These awkward postures either sustained or performed repeatedly may result in pain or sensitivity in the affected arm or arms.[7] Pain combined with acute weakening could indicate complete wear of the rotator cuff.

The symptoms, which can be severe at night, include pain, weakening, and discomfort in the shoulder. The diagnosis of rotator cuff tendinitis is usually made by physical examination and sometimes requires specific radiographic confirmation.

The typical symptoms of shoulder impingement syndrome include difficulty reaching up behind the back, pain with overhead use of the arm, and weakness of shoulder muscles.

Etiology

Anatomically, this group of muscles in the shoulder allows for a wide range of movement while maintaining the stability of the glenohumeral joint. If the stabilizing muscles are weakened or the repetitive movement exceeds the muscles' capacity to adapt to the load, the humerus is rolled forward, toward the acromion. This results in damage to the tendon between the muscles, resulting in pain (Fig 4-2).

This progressive situation causes gradual wear of the tendon that passes between the humerus and the acromion process. The glenohumeral joint is a very dynamic articulation, with ligaments and tendons, and a bursa, which is a synovial fluid that

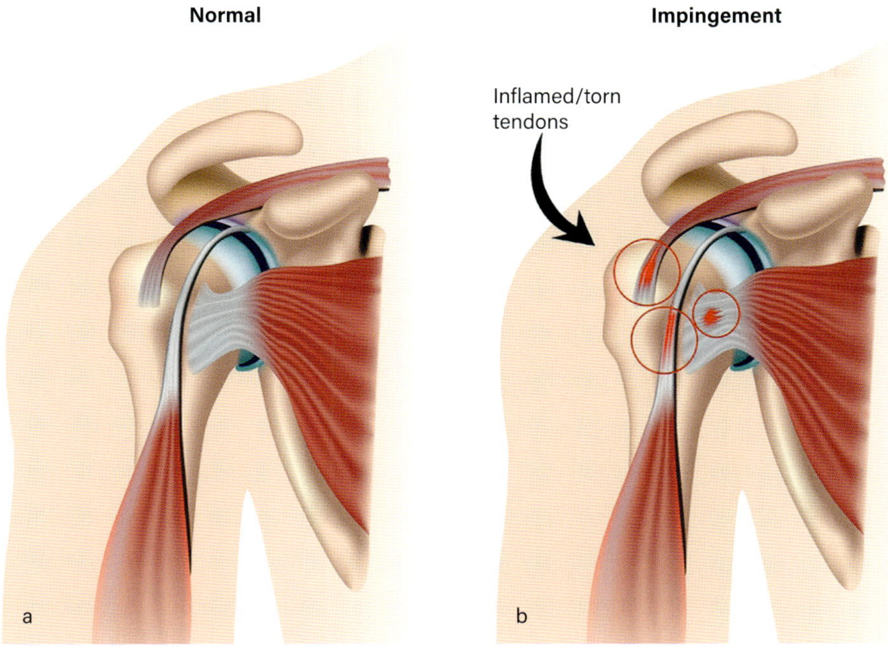

FIG 4-2 *(a)* Anatomy of the rotator cuff. *(b)* Rotator cuff impingement.

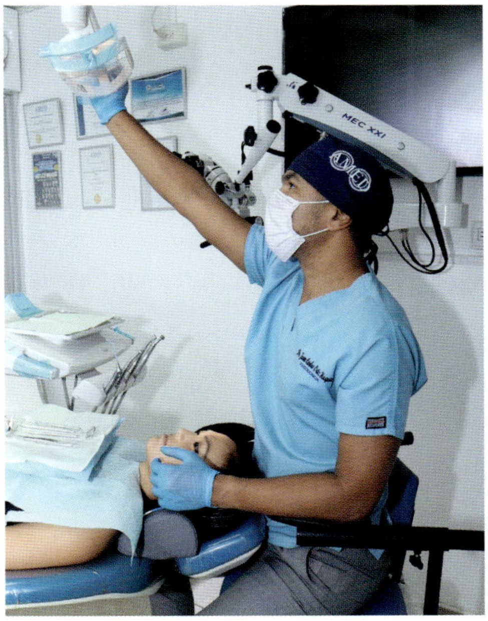

FIG 4-3 Elevation of the arm over the head frequently performed in dentistry.

acts as a cushion between tendons and other joint structures. Elevating the elbow to the shoulder is one of the principal ways to irritate the rotator cuff. This is how tendinopathy occurs involving the supraspinatus tendon (the tendon that helps raise the arm above the head) or any combination of the four rotator cuff tendons.

Rotator cuff tendonitis is an acute painful symptom in the tendons.[8] In dentistry, rotator cuff injury typically occurs due to microwear accumulation as a result of frequent awkward posture. Frequency of posture and movement is a risk factor for injury. Abducting and elevating the shoulder too often (Fig 4-3) results in instability and weakening of the stabilizing muscles and, eventually, complete wear of the of the rotator cuff tendon.

Neutral recommended shoulder abduction is 20 degrees, and motion beyond 30 degrees can promote blood flow to the supraspinatus tendon, which causes ischemia.[9] Positioning challenges and working habits with bad posture result in dentists abducting the arms. This is one of the reasons why positioning sequence must be respected during dental treatment. Positioning is everything.

Positioning is everything.

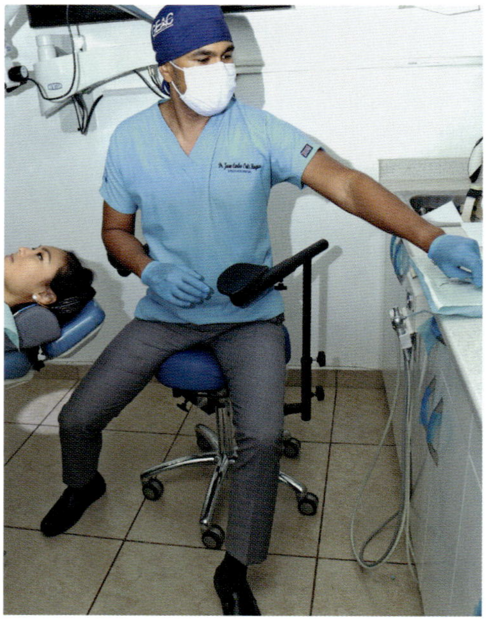

FIG 4-4 Torso rotation and arm abduction in dentistry without an assistant.

Shoulder/rotator cuff impingement generally occurs as a consequence of incorrectly positioning the patient in the dental chair. A classic example is when the patient's mouth is far from the operator's head; to reach the patient's mouth, the operator must extend their arms more than 25 degrees forward from the shoulder joint. Another very frequent cause is either not working with an assistant or working with an assistant who is not properly trained. If the instruments and equipment are not placed close enough to the operator or assistant's hands, it becomes necessary to extend the arms from the shoulder to reach these items (Fig 4-4). These are just some examples—any movement or posture that implies an excess of movement in that area places the dentist, hygienist, and assistant at risk of developing pain in this area.

Treatment and prevention

Treatment can range from anti-inflammatory medications for 1 to 2 weeks to modifying activities that exacerbate the problems. If the problem persists chronically, the tendon can actually tear in two, resulting in a rotator cuff tear that may require surgery.[10] Motion control and postural awareness are the best options to avoid awkward sustained postures of the shoulder joint area in order to protect it from wear and tear. Poor posture is an independent predictor of symptomatic and asymptomatic rotator cuff tear.[11]

Trapezius Myalgia

The upper trapezius is a large fan-shaped muscle that extends from the cervical to thoracic region on the posterior aspect of the neck and trunk and attaches onto the clavicle and scapula (see Fig 4-1b). Disorders in dentistry related to trapezius muscle overuse, repetitive work, forceful exertion, prolonged static posture, high intensity, and monotonous working tasks can result in a painful condition called *trapezius myalgia*.

Symptoms and etiology

The following are symptoms of trapezius myalgia:

- Sudden pain
- Muscle stiffness and spasms
- Tightness of the neck-shoulder complex
- Occipital headache
- Heaviness of the head
- Tenderness of the upper trapezius

Symptoms usually occur on the side holding the mirror or from where the soft tissue retraction is performed. Trigger points on these muscles can cause referred pain, which spreads to one of the sides of the neck, as well as headaches behind the eye.[12] The upper trapezius muscle is responsible for lifting the shoulders and rotating the head as well as supporting the weight of the arms, which increases the muscle tension in the neck and shoulders. Some studies have found that dentists are exposed to a high demand on the trapezius muscles bilaterally due to forward bending of the head.[13]

Systematic positioning is like a domino effect. Consider a patient positioned too high in the chair. This will result in the operator systematically raising the shoulders to allow them to work in the patient's mouth. Even if an optical microscope is used in this situation, the microscope will be placed too high, putting the operator's head into hyperextension and stressing the trapezius muscles to stabilize the neck.

Fatigue

Biomechanically, the requirement of a proper visual field into the oral cavity and nonsymmetric operator position puts the neck in a prolonged flexed forward and rotated posture, which can produce pain and muscle fatigue. Cognitive central fatigue due to excessive mental and emotional stress has also been found to cause contraction of this muscle,[14] which underscores the importance of incorporating stress management strategies. Scheduled ergo breaks and movement during dental tasks should be a regular part of the working day.

Prevention

Due to the nature of time and pressure in the dental profession, the organization of patient scheduling plays an important role in decreasing stress on the dentist and staff. Dentistry without an assistant results in wasted movements and increased stress.

Dentistry without an assistant results in wasted movements and increased stress.

Upper Limb Syndromes

There is no doubt that dental professionals are exposed to a wide variety of risks in the upper extremities. The nature of the tasks, performing them in reduced spaces, the need for precision on limited focal distances and field of view, overreaching for

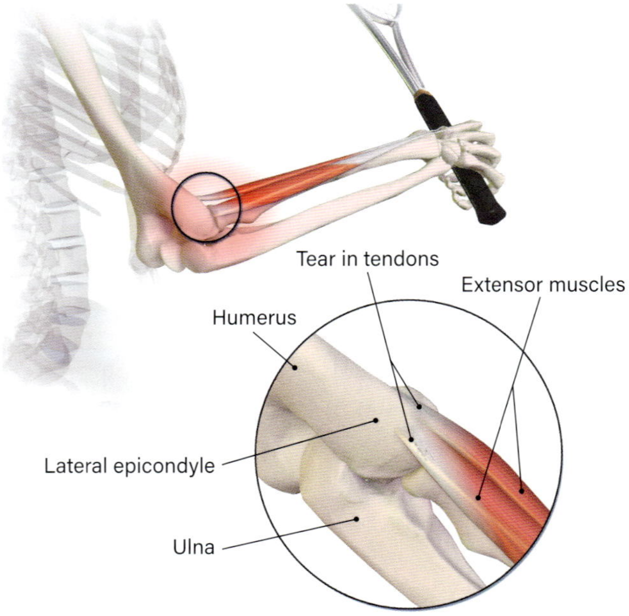

FIG 4-5 Lateral epicondylitis, also known as *tennis elbow*.

instruments and equipment, and dealing with situations of anxiety and constant stress all contribute to this risk.[8]

Cumulative trauma disorders are also frequent in the areas of the elbow joint, hand, and wrist. Those frequently encountered in dentistry include the following:

- Lateral epicondylitis
- Medial epicondylitis
- De Quervain's tenosynovitis
- Carpal tunnel syndrome

Cumulative trauma syndromes of the hand and wrist are present in between 23% and 40% of dental professionals and are more prevalent than in the general population due to applied forces, repetitive thumb abduction, sustained instrumental gripping, and awkward postures throughout the working day.[15–17] Postural awareness, properly gripping instruments, and programmed stretching of the elbow-wrist-hand joint are key to preventing these painful syndromes.

Lateral epicondylitis

Lateral epicondylitis, also known as *tennis elbow*, is a painful condition of the elbow caused by overuse. This is seen most often when the wrist extensors are contracted against opposing forces, such as when the dentist or hygienist extends the wrist out of the neutral position during repetitive tasks, such as pinching or gripping forces on the handpieces, forceps, mirror, or endodontic files for frequent or long time periods (Fig 4-5). The primary symptom is pain, especially during extensions of the wrist. In more advanced cases, there can also be pain during rest. The diagnosis can be made by physical examination.

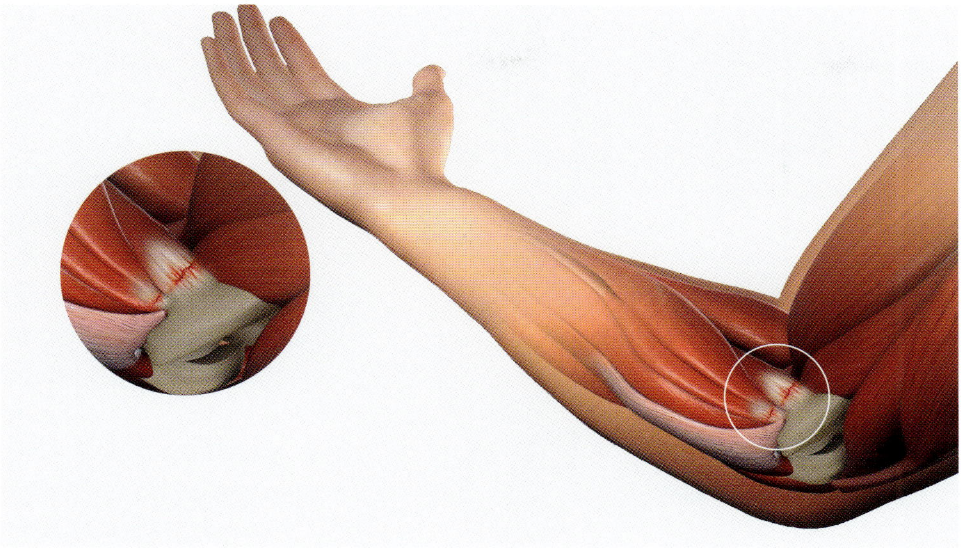

FIG 4-6 Medial epicondylitis, also known as *golfer's elbow*.

Medial epicondylitis

Medial epicondylitis, also called *golfer's elbow*, is a musculoskeletal disorder of the tendons that connect the forearm muscles to the inside elbow bone (Fig 4-6). It is an inflammation of the flexor wrist muscles that originate from the epicondyle medial of the elbow. Due to injury or irritation to the inside part of the elbow, where the medial epicondyle is located, structures can become swollen and painful. Generally, this occurs from any activity involving use of the arms or wrists.

Because this condition is caused by flexion of the wrist, particularly when combined with forced contractions against resistance, the pain is constant and exacerbated by wrist contractions. It has also been shown that many of the activities that cause tennis elbow can also cause golfer's elbow.[18]

The diagnosis is generally determined by a physical examination. Pain on palpation or flexion of the wrist is the most frequent symptom for diagnosis. Treatment includes modifying activities that exacerbate the problem, cold therapy, rest time for the limb, postural awareness, and physical therapy.

De Quervain's tenosynovitis

De Quervain's tenosynovitis, also associated with pain, is diagnosed when there is an inflammation of the extensors of the thumb and in the abductor tendons. It mostly occurs when we tilt the wrist in the direction of the thumb, what is known as *radial deviation*. Symptoms increase in the base of the thumb with increasing deviation, and sometimes pain can migrate to the extensor of the thumb and to the tendons and muscles of the forearm region.

The diagnosis is made by physical examination of the wrist in the radial deviation while the patient makes a fist around the thumb.[10] During this test, the patient typically reports severe pain in the tendons at the site of the affected finger. Rest time, stretching, cold compress, anti-inflammatory medication, and physical therapy with massages could be considered a therapeutic form of healing.

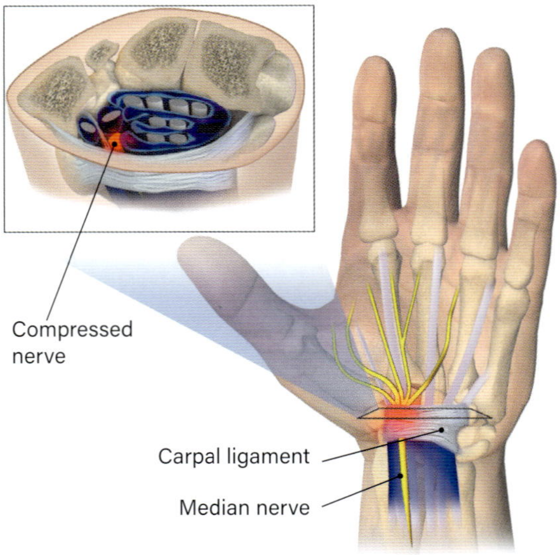

FIG 4-7 Anatomy of the carpal tunnel and carpal tunnel syndrome.

Carpal tunnel syndrome

Carpal tunnel syndrome is a common condition in the hand and arm area that occurs when the medial nerve is compressed in the carpal tunnel of the wrist, causing pain, numbness, and tingling in the hand and arm.[19] The carpal tunnel is a narrow passageway in the wrist, about an inch wide. The floor and sides of the tunnel are formed by small wrist bones called *carpal bones* (Fig 4-7). This syndrome is responsible for one of the most common hand surgeries performed in the United States.[20] Up to 71% of dentists suffer one or more symptoms of carpal tunnel syndrome, but only 7% are diagnosed.[21] According to the National Institute of Neurological Disorders and Stroke,[22] this disorder generally occurs in the dominant hand and most frequently in adults performing repetitive motions. According to some studies, women develop carpal tunnel syndrome three times more frequently than men.[22,23]

Up to 71% of dentists suffer from symptoms of carpal tunnel syndrome.

Because the origin of the problem is in the muscles and tendons that stabilize the arm during repetitive work, any compression on the medial nerve fibers can result in some symptoms of carpal tunnel syndrome in the hand.[22] In dentistry, there are two main situations that may produce this syndrome:

- *Repetitive hand use:* Repeating the same hand and wrist motions or activities over and over again for prolonged periods of time may cause pressure on the medial nerve in the wrist carpal tunnel area.
- *Hand and wrist position:* The activity of extreme flexion or extension of the hand and wrist for a prolonged period of time.

The National Institute of Neurological Disorders and Stroke recommends that treatments for carpal tunnel syndrome should begin as early as possible, under a doctor's direction.[22] (Underlying causes such as diabetes or arthritis should always be treated first.) Treatment depends on the stage of the disease and can be nonsurgical or surgical. Nonsurgical treatments include the following[22]:

- Splinting
- Avoiding activities that may provoke symptoms
- Over-the-counter drugs such as NSAIDs (nonsteroidal anti-inflammatory drugs)
- Prescription drugs such as corticosteroids
- Alternative therapies such as acupuncture, chiropractic treatment, and yoga

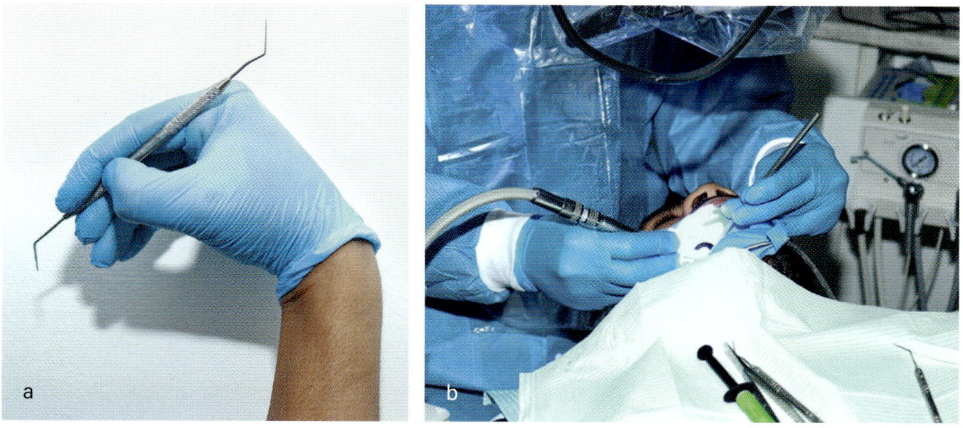

FIG 4-8 *(a)* Flexioned wrist-hand holding an instrument. This is a nonneutral wrist posture. *(b)* The wrist and hand are in a neutral position, aligned with the arm.

Prevention

The most important point is to avoid sustained flexion of the wrist. A knowledge of biomechanics and postural awareness can help with this. Working with the wrist inclined toward the little finger, known as *ulnar deviation*, also increases this pressure.[20] When scaling with ultrasound, working with a handpiece, using endodontic files, and holding instruments during dental work in general, the wrist should be kept straight (Fig 4-8). Think of the hand, wrist, and forearm as a single unit. The assistant can help by constantly observing the position of the wrist and alerting the operator when it is deviating from the neutral posture. In the long run, this will create the habit of postural awareness—not only of the wrist, but for other areas as well.

The use of finger rests has been suggested to reduce muscle fatigue and stress as well as to stabilize the instrument while performing dental scaling or other types of dental work.[24] Finger rest points—either intraoral or extraoral—can also be used to stabilize a mirror used for direct vision. This can help to reduce the grip strength of the thumb and muscle loads on the hand.[24] Extraoral fulcrums also facilitate neutral wrist posture and allow proper positioning for precise instrumentation.[25] A simple guide for neutral wrist posture is when the hand is in the orientation of thumb up and aligned with the forearm.

Some mistakes that promote wrist awkward posture include the following:

- Gripping the mirror near the glass area on the handle
- Positioning the mouth of the patient too close or too far away
- Working from the 9 o'clock position

In dentistry, gripping and pinching force is another risk factor to consider. Due to sustained grips of small instruments and prolonged uncomfortable postures for most of the day, pain in the hand, wrist, and forearm is prevalent.[26] About 23% to 40% of dentists suffer from hand and wrist pain.[24,27]

Conclusion

The functionality of the upper limb is interconnected. The correct use of each of the body segments that allow the development of work in dentistry obviously requires repeated movements and holding instruments or equipment for a long time. This is the clinical reality. However, maintaining healthy posture of the wrists (aligned with the forearm) as well as performing programmed stretching of the wrist flexors and extensors can help prevent the common syndromes associated with our daily work.

Most of these syndromes are preventable in dentistry by focusing on the way we use our body and interact with the instruments and equipment we use in the office. Sometimes, the technical nature of the profession requires putting prolonged static forces in nonneutral postures of the upper limbs, which makes prevention a challenge. However, the use of the dental microscope and the ergonomic stool could help in supporting the involved structures, and programmed stretching and simply being aware of neutral postures can make a big difference. We must remain motivated to protect ourselves from injury and take the right steps to work without pain.

References

1. Morse T, Bruneau H, Dussetschleger J. Musculoskeletal disorders of the neck and shoulder in the dental professions. Work 2010;35:419–429.
2. Rodiger A. How to Sit Your Body at Work: A Guide to Sitting at Your Workstation Based on the Alexander Technique. Indianapolis: Dog Ear, 2010.
3. Bansal A, Bansal P, Kaur S, Malk A. Prevalence of neck disability among dental professionals in North India. J Evol Med Dent Sci 2013;2:8782–8787.
4. Ariëns GA, Bongers PM, Douwes M, et al. Are neck flexion, neck rotation, and sitting at work risk factors for neck pain? Results of a prospective cohort study. Occup Environ Med 2001;58:200–207.
5. Morrison G. Workplace Ergonomics and Neck Pain. Spine-Health. https://www.spine-health.com/conditions/neck-pain/workplace-ergonomics-and-neck-pain. Accessed 11 March 2022.
6. Thornton LJ, Stuart-Buttle C, Wyszynski TC, Wilson ER. Physical and psychosocial stress exposures in US dental schools: The need for expanded ergonomics training. Appl Ergon 2004;35:153–157.
7. Saunders D, Saunders RL, Kraus SL, Woerman A. Evaluation, Treatment, and Prevention of Musculoskeletal Disorders. Philadelphia: Saunders, 1995.
8. Pollack-Simon R. All the Right Moves: The Definitive Guide for Integrating Dental Team Ergonomics. Tulsa, OK: Pennwell, 2002.
9. Karwowski W, Marras WS. The Occupational Ergonomics Handbook. Boca Raton, FL: CRC, 1999.
10. Valachi B. Practice Dentistry Pain-Free: Evidence-Based Strategies to Prevent Pain and Extend Your Career. Portland, OR: Posturedontics, 2008.
11. Yamamoto A, Takagishi K, Kobayashi T, et al. The impact of faulty posture on rotator cuff tears with and without symptoms. J Shoulder Elbow Surg 2015;24:446–452.
12. Donnelly JM, Fernández-de-las-Peñas C, Finnegan M, Freeman JL. Travell, Simons & Simons' Myofascial Pain and Dysfunction: The Trigger Point Manual, ed 3. Philadelphia: Wolters Kulwer, 2019.
13. Jonker D, Rolander B, Balogh I. Relation between perceived and measured workload obtained by long-term inclinometry among dentists. Appl Ergon 2009;40:309–315.
14. Westgaard RH. Effects of physical and mental stressors on muscle pain. Scand J Work Environ Health 1999;25(suppl 4):19–24.
15. Valachi B. Getting the Upper Hand on Pain: Preventing Hand and Wrist Pain Syndromes in Dental Professionals. https://dentalacademyofce.com/courses/1878/pdf/handandwristpain.pdf.pdf. Accessed 11 March 2022.
16. Hamann C, Werner RA, Franzblau A, Rodgers PA, Siew C, Gruninger S. Prevalence of carpal tunnel syndrome and median mononeuropathy among dentists. J Am Dent Assoc 2001;132:163–224.
17. Rucker LM, Sunell S. Ergonomic risk factors associated with clinical dentistry. J Calif Dent Assoc 2002;30:139–148.

18. Morrey BF, Sanchez-Sotelo J, Morrey ME. Morrey's The Elbow and Its Disorders, ed 5. Philadelphia: Elsevier, 2018.
19. Anto C, Aradhya P. Clinical diagnosis of peripheral nerve compression in the upper extremity. Orthop Clin North Am 1996;27:227–236.
20. Mackin EJ, Callahan AD, Skirven TM, Schneider LH, Osterman AL, Hunter JM. Rehabilitation of the Hand and Upper Extremity. St Louis: Mosby, 2002.
21. Rice VJ, Nindl B, Pentikis JS. Dental workers, musculoskeletal cumulative trauma, and carpal tunnel syndrome: Who is at risk? A pilot study. Int J Occup Saf Ergon 1996;2:218–233.
22. National Institute of Neurological Disorders and Stroke. Carpal Tunnel Syndrome Fact Sheet. https://www.ninds.nih.gov/Disorders/Patient-Caregiver-Education/Fact-Sheets/Carpal-Tunnel-Syndrome-Fact-Sheet. Accessed 11 March 2022.
23. Mackinnon SE, Novak CB, Landau WM. Clinical diagnosis of carpal tunnel syndrome. JAMA 2000;284:1924–1926.
24. Dong H, Barr A, Loomer P, Rempel D. The effects of finger rest positions on hand muscle load and pinch force in simulated dental hygiene work. J Dent Educ 2005;69:453–460.
25. Matsuda S, Pattison GL. Extraoral fulcrums: The essentials of using extraoral fulcrums for periodontal instrumentation. Dimens Dent Hyg 2004;2. https://dimensionsofdentalhygiene.com/article/extra-oral-fulcrums/. Accessed 4 June 2021.
26. Abbas SU. Pinch Force and Work-Related Musculoskeletal Disorders in Dental Professionals [thesis]. Farmington: University of Connecticut, 2004.
27. Alexopoulos EC, Stathi IC, Charizani F. Prevalence of musculoskeletal disorders in dentists. BMC Musculoskelet Disord 2004;5:16.

The Role of the Dental Assistant: Four-Handed Dentistry

5

The term *four-handed dentistry* was first recorded in 1960. Since then, this term has become widely used, and it refers to the active participation of a well-trained assistant next to the operator during all dental activities and procedures.[1] Four-handed work allows the operator to focus their efforts exclusively in the operative field, while the assistant handles the transfer of all necessary instruments to carry out the procedure.

Four-handed dentistry is what I call the "team systematic workflow approach." It is based on a set of principles that define the conditions under which efficiency can be attained in dental practice. Teamwork will guarantee the best performance within the office by the assistant and the operator. For this to occur, communication must be fluid between both, where the dentist must take the time necessary to train the assistant thoroughly so that there is a synergy of work.

Duties of the Dental Assistant

When the assistant stops performing the functions that allow the operator to focus solely and exclusively on the operative field of work, the work on the part of the operator becomes more demanding. The operator will perform many unnecessary movements that cause physical fatigue and mental stress. In addition, interruptions act as a distraction for the operator, which can have the further effect of lowering the quality of the dental procedure to be executed.

The assistant's primary operational tasks are to keep the mirror clean during active work by the dentist with the high-speed handpiece (cleaning any dirt, fog, or water that obstructs the visibility through the mirror by gently blowing air with the triple syringe softly; Fig 5-1), retracting soft tissue, rinsing and drying the field, transferring instruments and handpieces, and adjusting the light when working without a surgical light microscope.

Chapter objectives

- **Be aware of the correct position of the assistant**
- **Understand how the assistant should handle instruments**
- **Learn how to assist in the prevention of musculoskeletal pain in the assistant**
- **Utilize the types of delivery system that favor the development of adequate workflow**
- **Learn the basics of working with indirect vision (the mirror technique)**

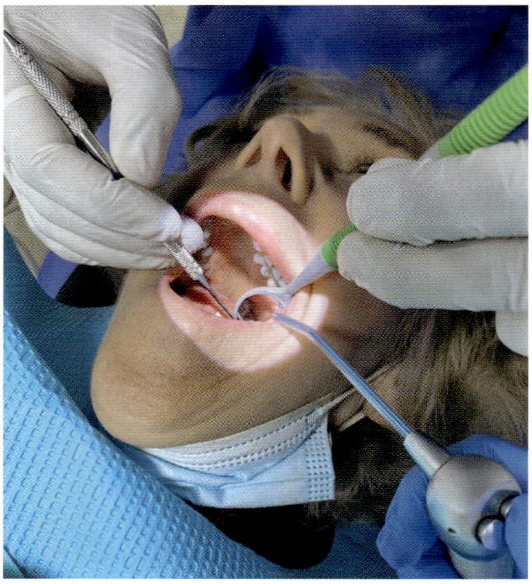

FIG 5-1 The assistant blows air with the triple syringe to keep clear visibility with the mirror and avoid interruptions for the operator.

In this cooperative process, there are several important principles that should be observed[2]:

- Equipment is ergonomically designed to minimize unnecessary motions.
- The operating team and patient are seated comfortably in ergonomically designed equipment.
- The dentist assigns all legally delegable duties to qualified auxiliaries based on guidelines.
- Patient treatment is planned in advance in a logical sequence.
- Motion economy is practiced.
- Preset trays are utilized.
- Safety procedures and standardized infection control procedures are implemented.

Four-handed dentistry is, ergonomically, the most favorable way to provide dental treatment.

The right investment in training and equipment for the dental assistant can bring productivity benefits, as well as job satisfaction and career longevity.[3] Four-handed dentistry is, ergonomically, the most favorable way to provide dental treatment because it minimizes undesirable motions for the entire work team and is one of the foundations of dental ergonomics (see chapter 1). Without an assistant, there will not be a fully ergonomic practice.

Posture of the Dental Assistant

While the dental assistant is key to improving productivity and decreasing stress for the dentist, the assistant can also suffer from musculoskeletal pain, mainly in the lower back.[4] Lack of education on ergonomics and inadequate design of office and delivery systems contribute greatly to the high rates of musculoskeletal disorders among dental assistants. Take the time to train your assistant so that the operatory becomes a stress-free, synergic environment.

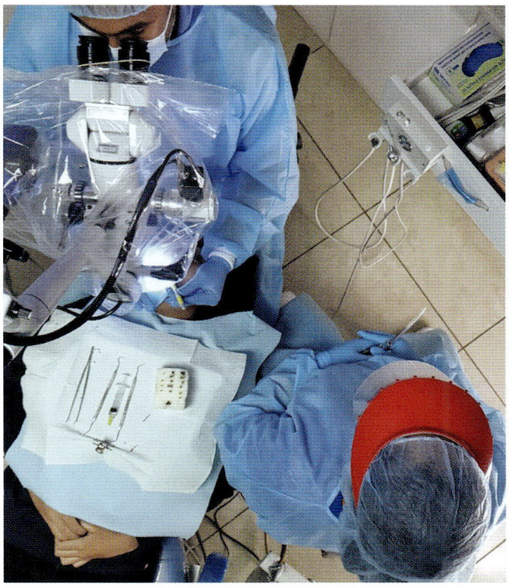

FIG 5-2 Ideal position of the assistant.

Just as the dentist should maintain neutral posture throughout work tasks, so too should the assistant. The same biomechanics and psychosocial stressors present for the dentist are also present for hygienists and assistants.[5] Because of this, assistants and hygienists should be included during ergonomic evaluations to establish the same work criteria from the postural, positional, and organizational points of view.

The following are some basic guidelines for neutral posture (see also chapter 3):

- From a side view, ears are vertically aligned with the shoulders and hips.
- From behind, the spine should be straight, without bending or twisting.
- The upper arm segments should not abduct more than 25 degrees, and the forward range must not exceed 20 degrees.[6]
- Shoulders should be relaxed to the sides, not elevated.
- Wrists should be kept as straight as possible, without ulnar deviation, flexion, or extension.

Remember that the greater the deviation from the neutral posture, the more tension will be generated in the muscles, tendons, ligaments, joints, and spinal discs.[3] Forward tilt or side twist postures are a powerful combination that explains why assistants also have a high risk of lower back pain, specifically if horizontal reaching positioning of instruments with constant or frequent use is not respected. The combination of nonergonomic office design and lack of ergonomic training for assistants is an obstacle to attaining the best ergonomic environment in the office.[7]

To avoid leaning forward and allow the maintenance of a neutral posture, the assistant should sit as close as possible to the dentist and to the patient's oral cavity. Ideally, they should sit with the left thigh parallel to the dentist's left shoulder and the patient's mouth; this way, the knees will bend toward the patient's head (Fig 5-2). Having a delivery system behind the patient will allow the assistant direct access to instruments, handpieces, and triple syringe and will prevent them from needing

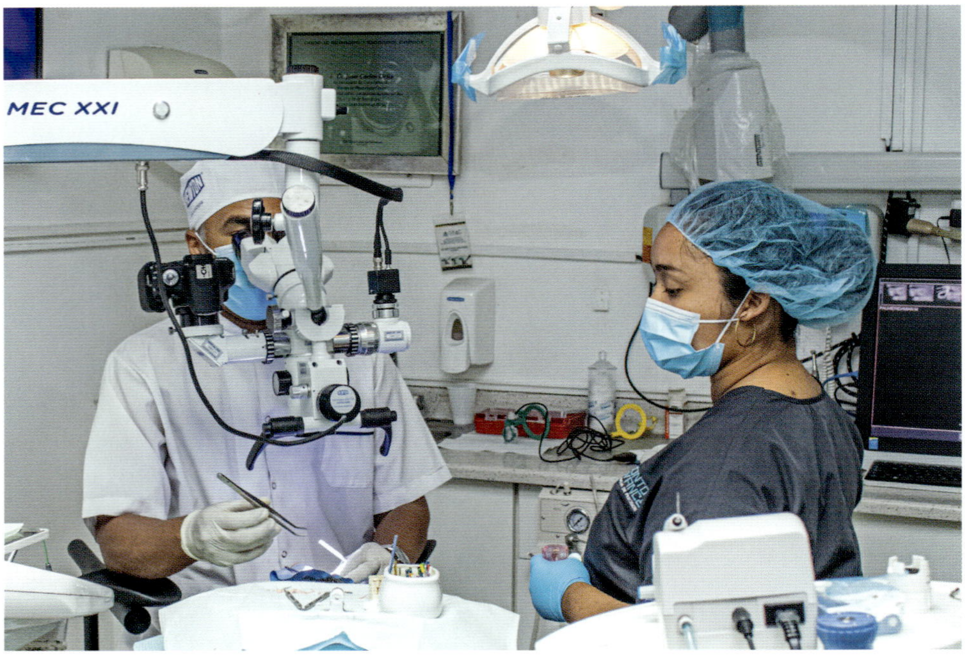

FIG 5-3 The assistant's eye height is at the same level as the dentist's.

to rotate the torso and tilt the upper body to pick up instruments and equipment. This is the ideal position for work with the optical microscope, with the dentist at 12 o'clock, because it does not interfere with the dentist's posture and movement.[8]

Another important consideration is the height of the assistant in the chair. They should be at the operator's eye level, or 3 to 5 inches higher to allow a viewing angle into the oral cavity. This allows the assistant to work with suction, anticipate the movements of the operator, and more precisely transfer instruments (Fig 5-3).

Six-handed dentistry

In microscope-enhanced dental practice used in complex endodontic surgeries or long sedation procedures, handling is required by both the dentist and assistants for greater visibility, allowing the operator to focus in the working field. In this case, a third set of hands becomes essential in retraction and preparation of materials. While the first clinical assistant remains engaged in the treatment at the operation site, the second clinical assistant anticipates the needs of both the operator and the primary assistant.[9]

Working Environment for Four-Handed Dentistry

Furniture and layout of the operatory

To maximize efficiency, the environment must be properly set up and prepared for comfortable movement by the working team. Equipment should be selected according to the working area of the assistant, next to the patient chair, because most of the movement of instruments and materials occurs in this area during the procedures (see Fig 5-2). Some dental chairs can provide better or worse environments for the assistant to reach. For example, dental units without spittoons allow the assistant to get closer and move freely toward the operator and the work area close to the patient's mouth. Box 5-1 demonstrates recommendations for a systematic workflow with four-handed dentistry.

BOX 5-1 Recommendations for a systematic workflow

Assistant positioning
- Left thigh parallel to the patient's left shoulder and mouth
- Suction, triple syringe, and an extra handpiece in front of the assistant and behind the patient
- If the delivery system is not behind the patient, consider a mobile cart or modifications to the existing mobiliary
- Eyes at the same level or slightly higher than the operator's

Workflow
- Prepare the trays beforehand for each patient depending on the procedure
- Provide scheduled breaks for the assistant to rest and stretch during the workday
- Manage horizontal working distances by placing constant-use items within 40 cm of the assistant's hands and frequent-use items within 50 to 55 cm
- During active work in the mouth, the assistant must keep the mirror clean and visible to avoid interruptions

Ergonomically speaking, the primary focus when choosing a dental unit must be the assistant. This will alleviate unnecessary motions of the dentist and provide accessibility to handpieces and other dynamic instruments that should be primary to the assistant and secondary to the operator. The main idea is that the operator focuses on the work area in the patient's mouth, minimizing their hand motions anywhere else. Everything that happens outside the patient's mouth must be handled by the assistant, guaranteeing both economy of movements for the operator, concentration on work, and proper workflow. If the dentist must be constantly reaching for things such as triple syringe or suction, this will cause interruptions, which will disrupt an efficient workflow and cause physical strain.[10] However, the position of a tool such as the high-speed handpiece, which will have constant and repeated use, must be located closer to the operator than the assistant.

The primary focus when choosing a dental unit must be the assistant.

The assistant's ergonomic stool also plays a crucial role in improving the posture of their back and allowing them to sit comfortably. The stool should have accessories such as lumbar supports and a footrest. The stool should be selected based on the anthropometrics and dimensions of the individual's body, customized for them.

The assistant cannot sit too close to the operator either; a position too close will cause the assistant's knees to collide with the dentist's, especially when the dentist is located at the 11 o'clock or 12 o'clock position or if one of them has long legs. A position that guarantees both the assistant and operator will be close to the patient's mouth is the zipper position, in which the legs are intertwined (Fig 5-4). This position could be very useful when the dentist is located between 9 and 11 o'clock, whether or not the microscope is being used.

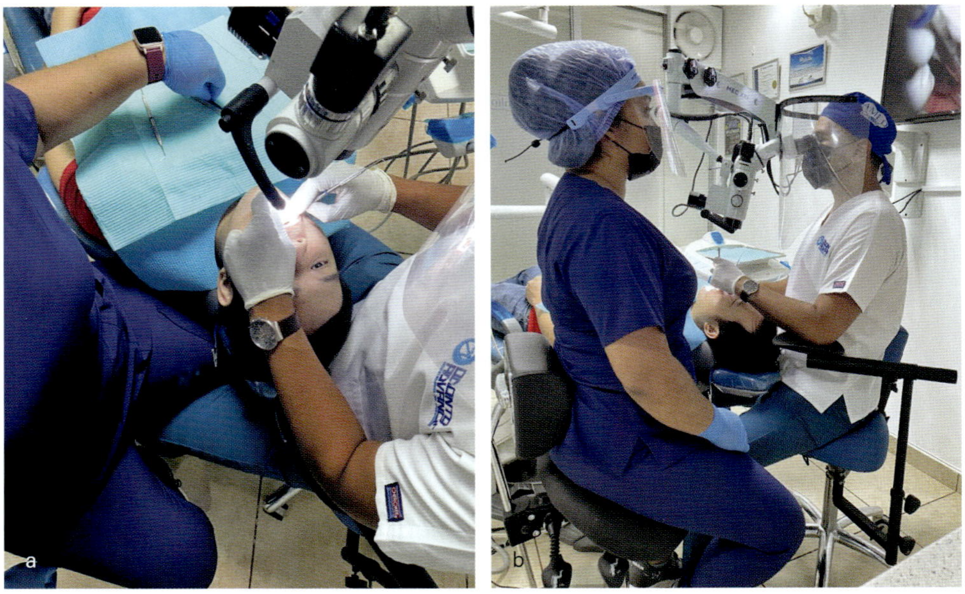

FIG 5-4 *(a and b)* The legs of the assistant and operator are in a zipper position. Again, note the eye level of the assistant.

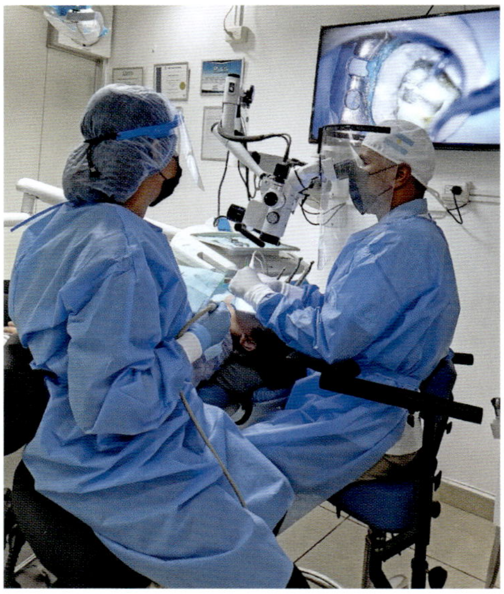

FIG 5-5 The live images captured through the microscope provide the assistant with an excellent view of the procedure, allowing them to anticipate the operator's movements and needs.

Dental practice with a microscope has the advantage of strategically placing screens to allow the assistant to see the entire procedure. This will allow the assistant to learn how the procedure works and help them to anticipate the operator's movements and manage work protocols (Fig 5-5). All this will affect the quality of the final dental work.[11]

Positioning of tools

One of the primary goals of ergonomics is to allow the operator to focus on the working field without interruption. The teamwork provided by the assistant's participation in four-handed dentistry makes this possible because the motions of each person can be planned in the most efficient way (Fig 5-6).

All the instruments must be within a radius of 50 cm from the assistant to be properly transferred to the dentist's hands, and constant-use instruments should be within 40 cm.[12,13] This enables the dental team to have everything within reach, which facilitates efficient and high-quality dental treatment. The use of carts, trays, and adjustable mobiliary can help the assistant organize the instruments and place items within horizontal reaching distances, allowing for efficiency during the working time with the dentist.

Within our daily clinical practice, we organize the work according to the principle of the triangle of influence. The three components that make up the triangle

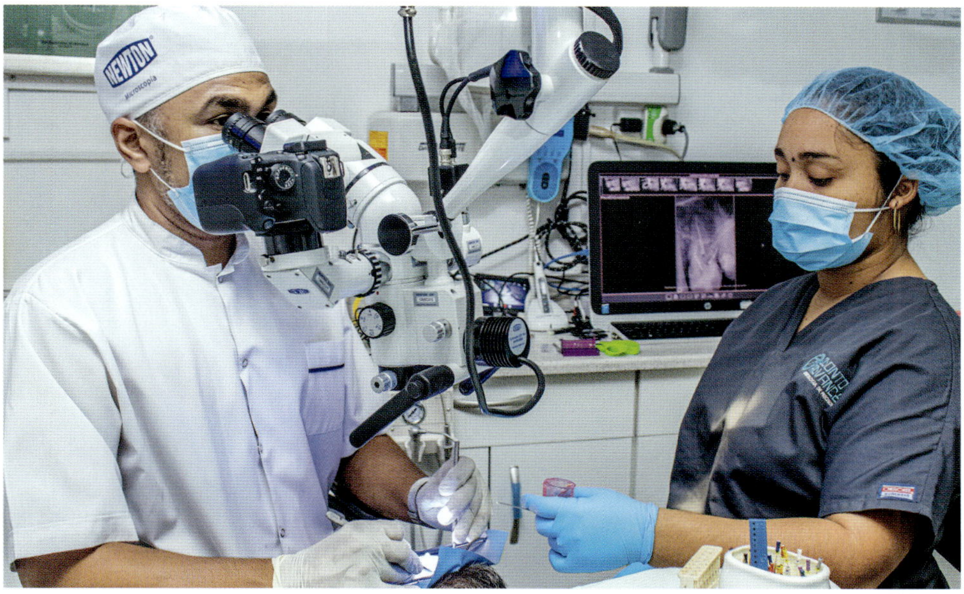

FIG 5-6 The assistant can easily transfer constant-use instruments to the operator in four-handed dentistry.

include *(1)* the operator, *(2)* the assistant, and *(3)* the set of supplies, instruments, and equipment (Fig 5-7). In the center of the triangle is the patient's mouth. In some instances, if it is acceptable to the patient, a tray can be placed on their chest for the most constant-use instruments. Manufacturers have created trays specifically for this purpose (eg, Bodytray, InterM) that are designed to be comfortable for the patient and stable to prevent instruments from slipping or moving even if the patient moves.

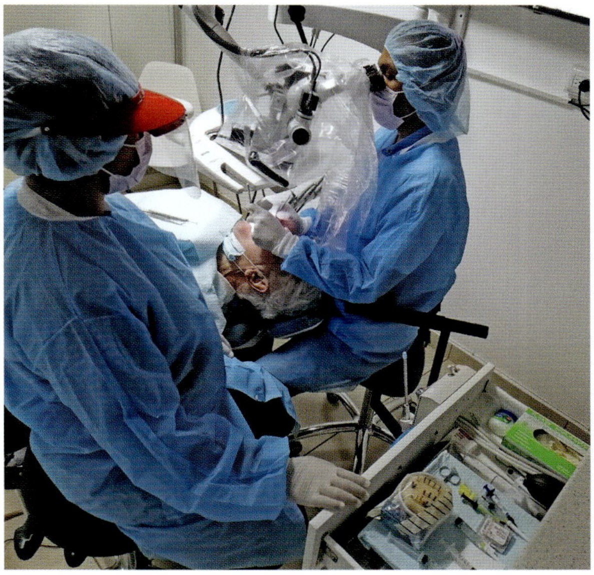

FIG 5-7 Triangle of influence: operator, assistant, and equipment, with the patient in the center.

The assistant must also consider the direction in which the instrument transfers to the operator. For example, the operator's hands and fingers will be positioned differently depending on the area of the mouth being worked on. The instrument should be handed off in a way that will follow the working direction, preventing the operator from needing to interrupt their work by changing the direction of the instrument. The handpieces are generally located on the operator's side, and an easy way to reduce motions by the operator is to take the handpiece, bring it to working position, and have the assistant change the burs without the operator removing their eyes from the working field (either naked-eye, with loupes, or with the microscope; Fig 5-8).

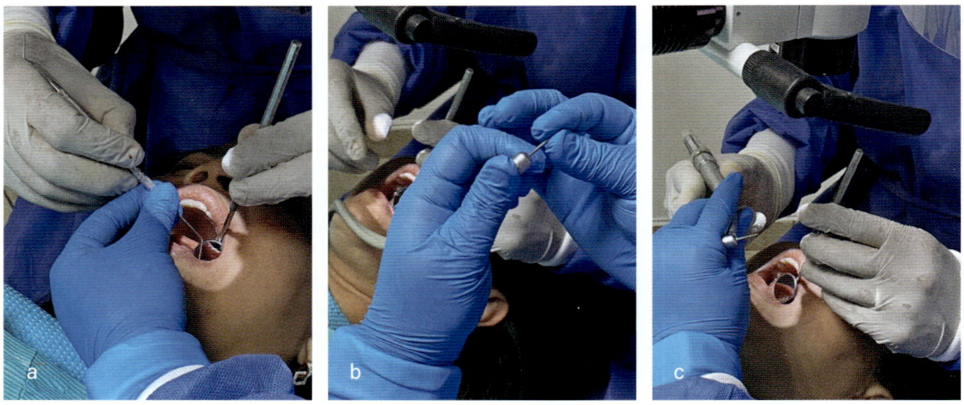

FIG 5-8 *(a)* The handpiece is transferred by the operator to the assistant's hands. *(b)* The assistant changes the bur. *(c)* The assistant delivers the handpiece back to the dentist's hands.

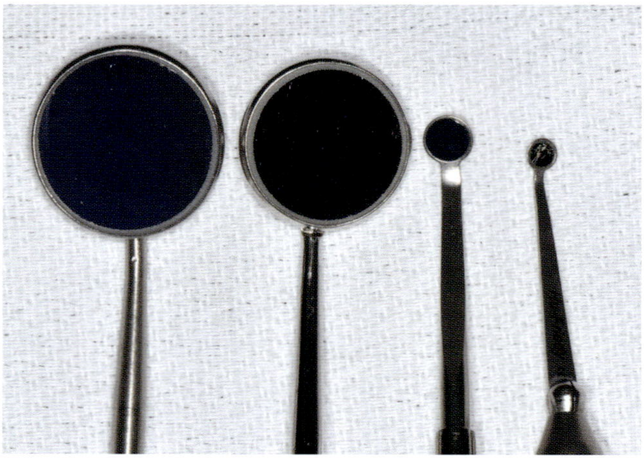

FIG 5-9 Different mirror sizes are available to improve visual access in the oral cavity and for use with the microscope.

Working with Indirect Vision: Mirror Technique

Using the mirror may have a major ergonomic impact due to the aid it provides for the position of the trunk and neck. Dentists who regularly use indirect vision tend to have fewer headaches and less neck and shoulder pain.[14] Also, it has been shown that bending to the side or rotating the neck more than 15 degrees for many hours can cause cervical spine damage, and this is typical head rotation when working without indirect vision or without an optical microscope.[15] The use of the dental mirror increases vision and contributes to the maintenance of neutral posture in the back and neck by reducing flexion in these body parts.[16]

The ideal grip should be in the middle third of the mirror handle using the thumb, index, and middle fingers so you can have a firm grip and rotate the mirror in all directions.

There are different mirror sizes with microscope magnifications to provide better access in difficult areas and manage procedures like difficult tooth preparation or accessing the apex of a root in apical surgery (Fig 5-9). The way to hold the mirror to enhance its use is also important—more so when we use the surgical microscope, which happens in almost 100% of procedures no matter which quadrant we are working on. The ideal grip should be in the middle third of the mirror handle using

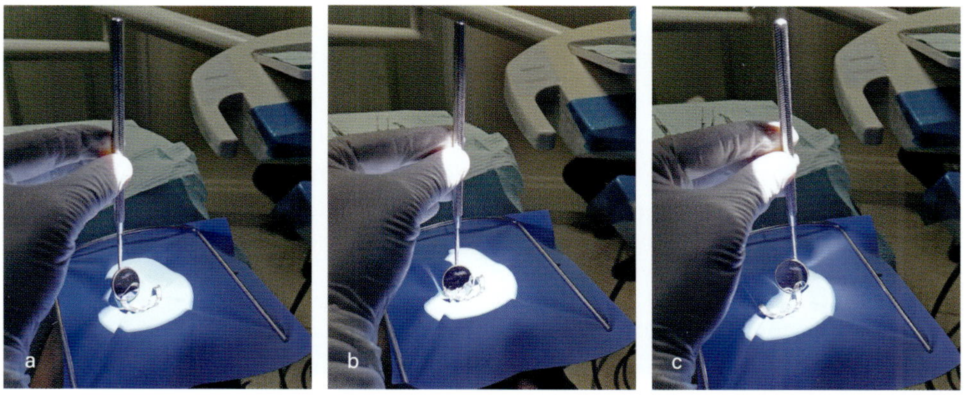

FIG 5-10 *(a)* Gripping the mirror comfortably to allow for easy movement. *(b and c)* This allows for rotation in either direction to provide visual information on different angles of the tooth.

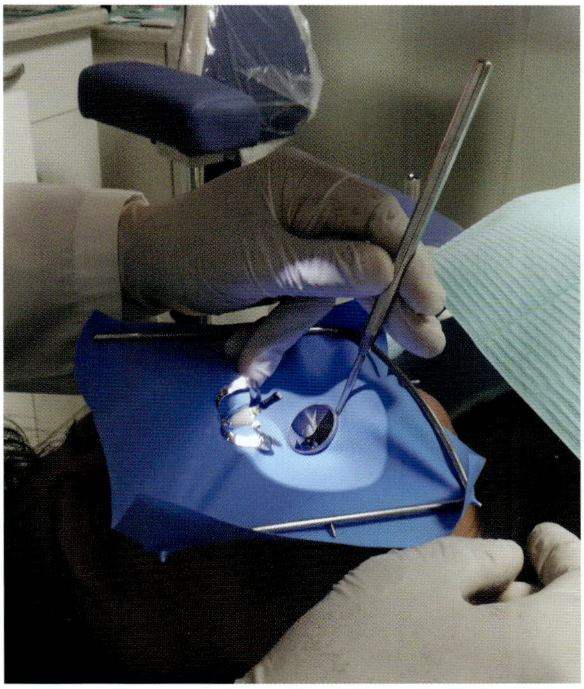

FIG 5-11 Mirror handling for indirect vision. Note how the operator's ring finger is stabilized against the patient's teeth.

the thumb, index, and middle fingers so you can have a firm grip and rotate the mirror in all directions (Fig 5-10). This type of grip will allow you to see the four surfaces of the tooth in all four quadrants of the mouth. The ring finger should function as an anchor or support against the adjacent teeth to provide stability (Fig 5-11). This is also very useful when taking optical microscope photographs to avoid mirror vibration and allow the image to be focused, not blurry. Also, gripping the handle without a supporting fulcrum point can be helpful in specific cases, such as in difficult access areas during diagnosis, while actively working with the handpiece or endodontic files, or in surgical procedures.

During our hands-on trainings, we have concluded that the proper use of the mirror in indirect vision closes the total ergonomics circuit when working with the microscope, because the skill allows the operator to maintain a suitable posture from the most neutral and symmetric position. Simple rotational movements with the mirror allow the operator to work actively on all tooth surfaces, both deep within the tooth and at complex localization angles such as the distolingual angle during the cutting of a mandibular molar or in restorative disciplines where the visual requirements are more dynamic than in endodontics. In naked-eye dentistry, managing indirect vision will keep the operator from side bending or forward leaning by keeping the focus on the mirror and not directly on the mouth, which has a positive impact on working posture.[17]

A suggestion from my experience to prevent bad posture both in dentistry with the naked eye and with magnification of any kind is to *(1)* use the mirror most of the time for indirect vision, *(2)* maintain an adequate positioning at 12 o'clock or as close to 12 o'clock as possible, and *(3)* manage the movements of the patient's head in order to obtain the best viewing angle rather than moving your own head and body to gain that visual access (see chapter 3).

Conclusion

Four-handed dentistry is one of the foundations of dental ergonomics. Having an assistant to hand you tools and help with your tasks is key to avoiding the muscle movements that will cause fatigue and cumulative trauma disorders. It will also help you to maintain neutral posture. The assistant should be properly trained and systematically positioned not only to provide maximum benefit to the operator, but also so that they too can maintain proper posture and avoid disorders. The dentist and assistant should sit close together (but not so close as to result in collisions) so tools can easily be handed from one to the other, and with the delivery system in easy reach of the assistant without requiring awkward reaching, twisting, or bending movements. Proper use of a dental mirror will also minimize uncomfortable movements.

References

1. Chasteen JE. Four-Handed Dentistry in Clinical Practice. St Louis: Mosby, 1978.
2. Finkbeiner BL. Are you ready to switch to four-handed dentistry? Dentistry IQ. https://www.dentistryiq.com/practice-management/staffing/article/16348394/are-you-ready-to-switch-to-fourhanded-dentistry. Accessed 24 March 2022.
3. Valachi B. The Ergonomics of Dental Assisting: Preventing and Managing Work-Related Pain. Annapolis, MD: American Dental Assistants Association, 2016.
4. Mulimani P, Hoe VC, Hayes MJ, Idiculla JJ, Abas AB, Karanth L. Ergonomic interventions for preventing musculoskeletal disorders in dental care practitioners. Cochrane Database Syst Rev 2018;10:CD011261.
5. Warren N. Causes of musculoskeletal disorders in dental hygienists and dental hygiene students: A study of combined biomechanical and psychosocial risk factors. Work 2010;35:441–454.
6. Chaffin DB, Andersson GBJ, Martin BJ. Occupational Biomechanics, ed 4. Hoboken, NJ: John Wiley & Sons, 2006.
7. Ohlendorf D, Erbe C, Nowak J, et al. Constrained posture in dentistry: A kinematic analysis of dentists. BMC Musculoskelet Disord 2017;18:291.
8. Blanc D, Farre P, Hamel O. Variability of musculoskeletal strain on dentists: An electromyographic and goniometric study. Int J Occup Saf Ergon 2014;20:295–307.
9. Dalai DR, Bhaskar DJ, Agali CR, Gupta V, Singh N, Bumb SS. Four handed dentistry: An indispensable part for efficient clinical practice. Int J Adv Health Sci 2014;1:16–20.
10. Bramson JB, Smith S, Romagnoli G. Evaluating dental office ergonomic. Risk factors and hazards. J Am Dent Assoc 1998;129:174–183.
11. Van As GA. The use of extreme magnification in fixed prosthodontics. Dent Today 2003;22(6):93–99.
12. Finkbeiner BL. Selecting equipment for the ergonomic four-handed dental practice. J Contemp Dent Pract 2001;2:44–52.
13. Pheasant S, Haslegrave CM. Bodyspace: Anthropometry, Ergonomics and the Design of Work, ed 3. Boca Raton, FL: Taylor and Francis, 2006.
14. Lehto TU, Helenius HY, Alaranta HT. Musculoskeletal symptoms of dentists assessed by a multidisciplinary approach. Community Dent Oral Epidemiol 1991;19:38–44.
15. Rundcrantz BL, Johnsson B, Moritz U. Occupational cervico-brachial disorders among dentists. Analysis of ergonomics and locomotor functions. Swed Dent J 1991;15:105–115.
16. Jeong YJ, Choi JS. The effect of indirect vision skills on head and shoulder posture amongst Korean dental hygienists. Eur J Dent Educ 2020;24:17–25.
17. Garcia PPNS, Pugliesi PMS, Wajngarten D, Neves TDC, Pazos JM, Dovigo LN. Development and assessment of an indirect vision training programme for operatory dentistry: Effects on working posture. Eur J Dent Educ 2022;26:36–44.

6

Ergonomic Dental Equipment

Selecting the Best Ergonomic Equipment

The dental equipment that is used every day and the way in which it is used directly affect the ergonomic position of the operator, assistant, and patient. Selecting the right ergonomic equipment that fits your body is an important consideration for musculoskeletal health in order to work comfortably. The most important element for the dentist is the stool—this is used more often and for longer than any other element.

For new dentists, equipment is one of the most important investments they will make in their career. As mentioned in previous chapters, many dentists suffer from some musculoskeletal disorder during dental school.[1] This is in part because institutional equipment is purchased considering financial concerns rather than ergonomic design. The ergonomic design of dental products has changed over the years thanks to advances in the knowledge of the correct sitting postures and four-handed dentistry. For example, having a stool with an adjustable height rather than a standard height will make a significant difference. The ability to customize your stool to your body height is one way to promote working in a healthy environment; it's the same as selecting the right tool for a given procedure. Comfort and adjustment to our physical and technical needs is an important consideration when choosing the tools and equipment we use.

Chapter objectives

- **Understand the functions of the operator's stool, including proper back and arm support, to allow you to work in neutral posture**
- **Recognize that patient dental chairs often are not designed for the operator to get close to the patient's mouth**
- **Understand the advantages and disadvantages of different dental chair delivery systems to allow the best choice to be made for your practice**
- **Consider the best layout for the assistant to efficiently reach elements such as suction and triple syringe, whether this includes modifying or improving the current operatory or making new purchases**

When patient chairs are purchased, the dentist often makes mistakes such as not considering the size of the operatory or focusing on patient comfort rather than operator comfort. Fortunately, the design of dental equipment is starting to move toward a more ergonomic design for the operator. However, an essential quality for ergonomic equipment is that it be adjustable to customize to the individual. Many designs may be labeled as "ergonomic," but this label becomes meaningless if the characteristics are only beneficial for someone with specific body dimensions. There is no "one size fits all" when choosing working tools.[2]

When acquiring new equipment or modifying the equipment you already have, the following factors should be considered for an efficient and ergonomic dental practice:

- The anthropometric and dimensional measurements of each individual
- The dimensions of the operatory
- The adjustability of the equipment or mobiliary that is already in the office

As discussed in chapter 5, four-handed dentistry is fundamental to ergonomic dental practice. Therefore, equipment should be selected with four-handed dentistry in mind. The team cannot successfully practice four-handed dentistry if there are obstructions inside the operatory, if the mobiliary cannot be reached by the assistant, or if the dental chair does not allow the dentist, hygienist, or assistant to reach the patient comfortably. A larger perspective that includes the whole picture should be considered.[3]

The most important factor when selecting any dental equipment is adjustability.

Investing in ergonomic changes to the office does not require thousands of dollars for renovation or products. Solutions can be as simple as positioning the patient differently, investing in an ergonomic operator stool or an ergonomic cushion for the seat, moving the patient in the chair, training the staff, and making minimal modifications to the equipment we already have. These are all changes that involve minimal expense and are supported by the advice of designers and professional ergonomists.

The most important items to consider from an ergonomic standpoint include the following:

- Operator's stool
- Patient chair and delivery system
- Fixed or mobile cabinetry
- Mobiliary and furniture

Operator's Stool

From an ergonomic point of view, the operator's stool is the most important chair in the office. Patients come and go, but the dentist, hygienist, and assistant spend hours and hours on the stool. The fact that we probably spend more time in contact with the stool than in our own beds should be more than enough motivation to learn the properties of an ergonomic stool and incorporate them into the office. The long-term health of the dentist depends on an appropriate stool.

While working, support from the backrest of a standard operator stool is usually not used because of positional challenges, bad sitting posture, or a poor design. Improving how you sit entails an appropriate knowledge of the features a stool should have, proper adjustment, proper selection of the seat, and understanding the differences of each seat, including shape, tilting properties, height adjustment, armrest dimensions, armrest adjustment, backrest mechanisms, backrest shape, and dimensions. Specific training to strengthen certain back muscles, such as the erector spinae (long muscles on each side of the spine) and the multifidus muscle (small muscles located near the spine, deep in the lower back), and use of the appropriate working distance and declination angle of the magnification instrument are some of the principal considerations to help the muscles and prevent fatigue.

The most important characteristics of the ergonomic stool include the following:

- Seat
- Backrest
- Armrest
- Height

Ideally, these features should be adjustable to customize to an individual's specifications. The stool should only need to be adjusted one time if used by only one operator. The stool should be adjusted to the following specifications:

- Your feet are resting comfortably on the floor or on a footrest (Fig 6-1).
- Your hips are higher than your knees (Fig 6-2).
- There is a gap of 2 to 4 inches between the back of your knees and the front edge of the chair when your back is against the chair (Fig 6-3).
- The curve of the backrest fits into and contacts the deepest part of the curve in your lumbar spine (Fig 6-4).
- The armrests are placed at elbow height when your arms are relaxed (Fig 6-5).
- The armrests do not interfere with access to the patient's mouth.

Every human body is different, with its own characteristics and anthropometric measurements. Not all models of stool will fit each person. Ideally, the stool should be tried out and adjusted to the specific user before it is purchased. Because this is not always possible or because stools may be shared among multiple operators, adjustability is crucial (Fig 6-6). There are chairs on the market that do not allow for adjustment of height, armrests, or backrests, and this limits their applicability.

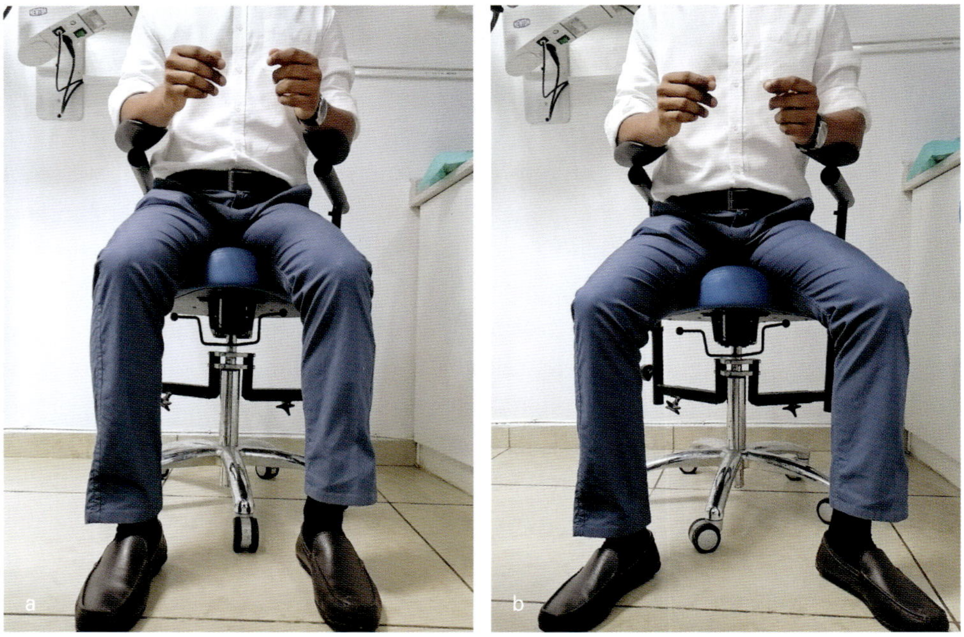

FIG 6-1 *(a)* Rest your feet comfortably on the floor in line with your knees and thighs. *(b)* If your feet are too far apart, place them in a frontal direction aligned with your knees.

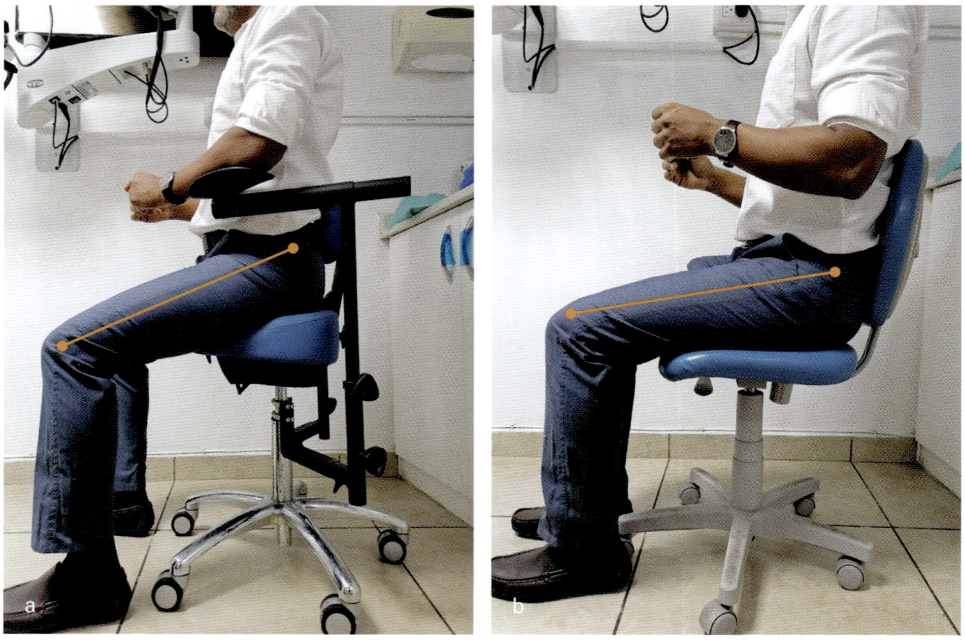

FIG 6-2 *(a)* The height and features of the stool seat should promote placement of the pelvis that is higher than the knees. *(b)* If the stool seat is too low, it should be raised.

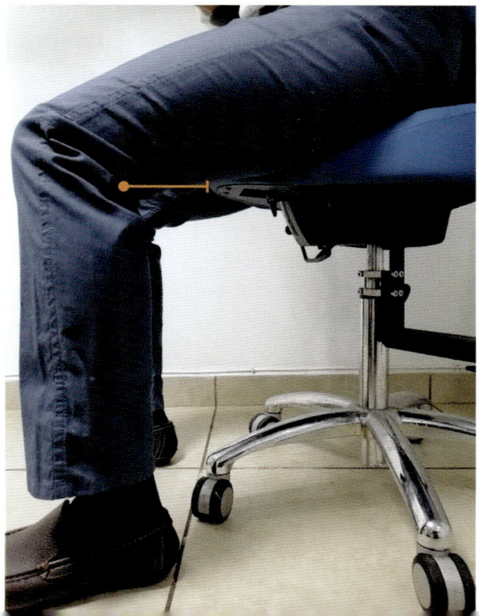

FIG 6-3 The seat pan of the stool should allow enough space for three finger-widths of distance between the end of the seat and the back of the knees.

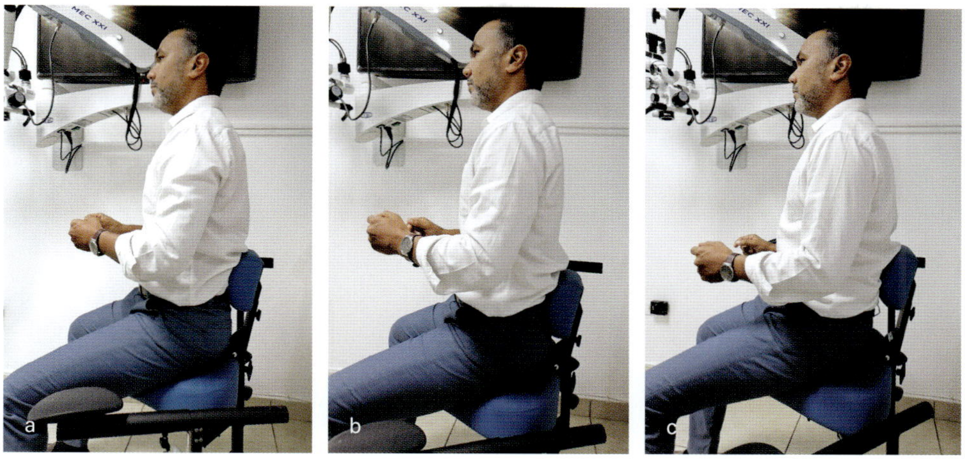

FIG 6-4 *(a)* The best way to promote lumbar protection is to adjust the backrest of the stool into the concave area of the lumbar spine. *(b)* The backrest is too low and does not support the concavity of the lumbar spine. *(c)* The backrest is too high and must be adjusted lower to provide proper support.

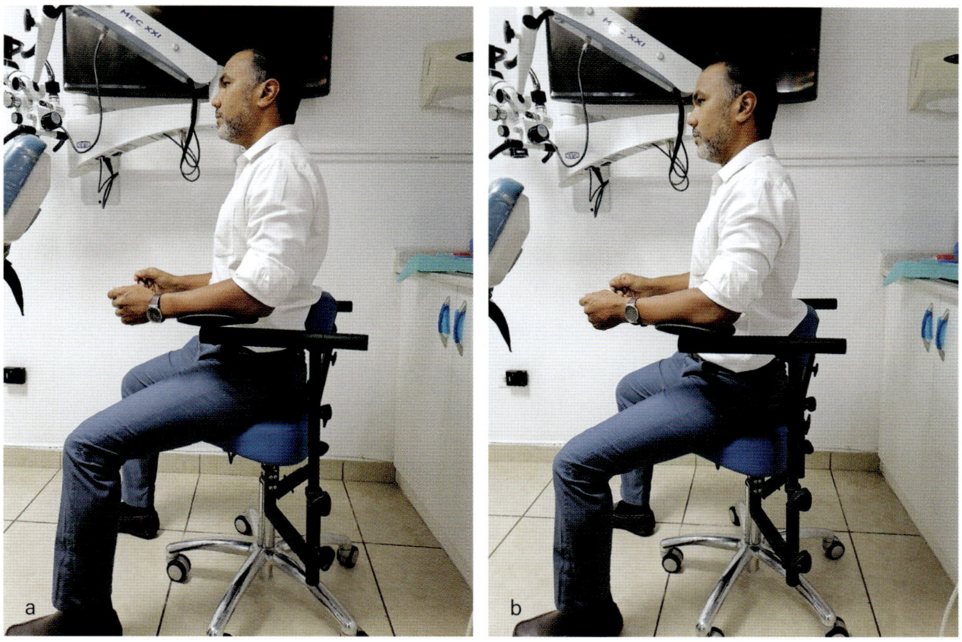

FIG 6-5 *(a)* Arm support is adjusted so the elbows are relaxed on both sides of the body. *(b)* If the armrests are too high, the shoulders become elevated, increasing tension on the shoulder joints.

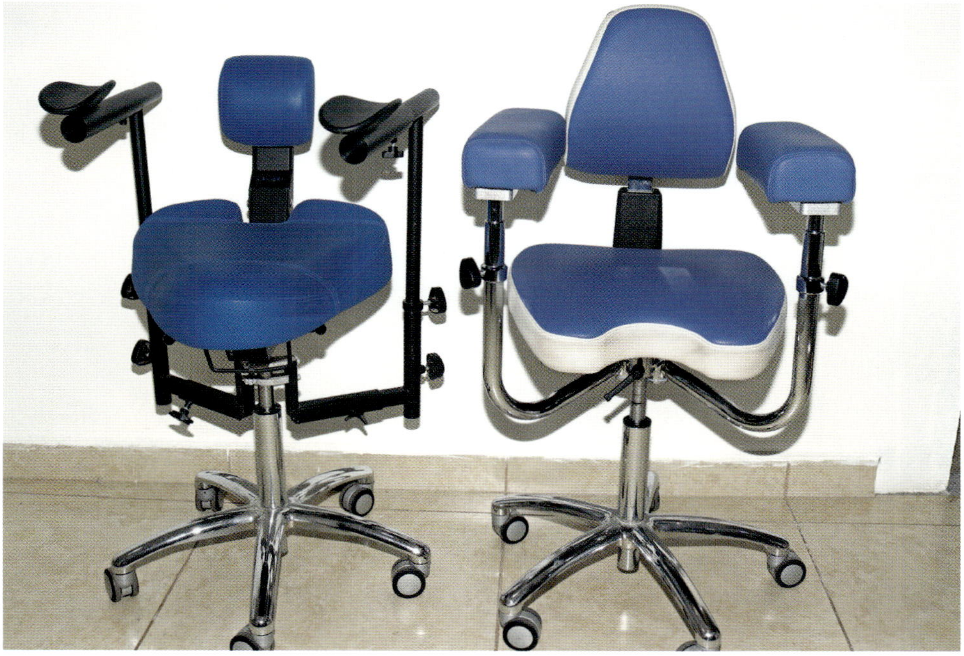

FIG 6-6 Examples of ergonomic stools. These are designed to allow neutral sitting posture, and the seat and arm height are adjustable.

The more neutral the pelvic position is, the more balanced the spinal curves will be, and the less tension will be generated in the back, neck, and shoulders.

Seat

The seat greatly affects the position of the pelvis, which is the basis of sitting posture. The more neutral the pelvic position is, the more balanced the spinal curves will be, and the less tension will be generated in the back, neck, and shoulders.

The operator must rest their feet on the floor and sit correctly. This means distributing the body weight on the stool. By sitting correctly, we provide a reference to the legs, back, and arms (if the armrest is used) to balance and give stability to the body. Keeping your feet flat on the floor without overusing them will decrease the chance of pushing and pulling the lower back muscles. This position allows the back to work more smoothly, improves breathing, and contributes to a lengthening and widening of the back throughout the upper body.[4]

We have commonly been taught to sit in flat seats with thighs parallel to the floor or with hips at a 90-degree angle to the legs in an L-shape. While performing relaxed seated work, this design may be tolerable; however, it becomes problematic when it is necessary to lean forward. The combination of leaning forward with the thighs parallel to the floor causes the pelvis to rotate backward and results in flattening of the lumbar curve.[5] As described in chapters 2 and 3, flattening the lumbar curve is harmful to the muscles of the back and discs of the spine.[6] The pelvis turns backward and causes a flattening in the lumbar curve because each spinal curve affects the ones above and below it: The flattened lumbar curve causes a reciprocal forward movement of the head, like a domino effect. In this position, the operator's spine provides very little support, and the body is held up by soft tissues from the spinal column, which easily gets fatigued with time.

Numerous studies report that the optimal working sitting position is with the hips higher than the knees. As the angle of the hips to the legs increases, muscle activity in the lower back is decreased, as is pressure on the discs. This requires a type of seat with a design that allows a slight downward tilt or saddle. The combination of a well-designed ergonomic operator stool and an understanding of the laws of biomechanics in relation to seated postures is fundamental to practicing ergonomic dentistry.

Seat depth

Seat depths range from 15 to 25 inches. When sitting to the edge of the seat and in contact with the backrest, there should be a space of at least three finger-widths between the edge of the seat and the back of the knee (see Fig 6-3). The seat should support two-thirds of the thighs. It is common to have stools with too much depth, which puts pressure on the thighs, reducing blood flow.

Seat width

The width of the seat must be such that it supports the operator entirely. Consideration should be given to the fact that deep seating and widths require more space around the patient chair to allow maneuverability. This is also why it is important to try the stool before making the purchase; body measurements are different among different people.

Seat contour

The contour of the chair has a great impact on comfort and support. The front edge must be padded and have a gradual downward slope. This feature is especially important when sitting with your thighs tilted down to reduce pressure on their blood vessels.

Seat pan tilting mechanism

Spinal loading and paraspinal muscle activities are reduced when sitting with adequate lumbar support on a seat pan that tilts. These are the two main features of an ergonomic stool to consider when making the purchase. A slight inclination of the seat pan between 5 and 15 degrees downward facilitates the natural lumbar curve in the lower back and decreases spinal load. However, a slope of more than 15 degrees seems to be counterproductive for the lower back.[7]

Seat texture

The seat material must be textured to prevent slipping when the operator leans down. Materials such as leather are modern and neat, unlike synthetics, which can be slippery and compromise the ergonomic benefits of the chair.[2]

Hydraulic controls

Control levers for easy adjustment are currently considered a standard feature for most chairs.

Saddle stool

The saddle stool is a newer concept in the design of seat pans in the dental industry. It promotes a neutral pelvic position by sloping the thighs downward more than the conventional seats, placing the hip at an angle of 125 degrees, almost like halfway between sitting and standing.[8,9] Some so-called "true" saddle stools can be found on the market. These are usually found without a backrest and with a split seat pan to provide more comfort to male users. One of the main disadvantages of this stool is that users—particularly men—can get some extra pressure in the peritoneal area, and no backrest is usually offered. Special attention should be placed when using the saddle stool in operators with hyperlordosis because it opens the hip angle more, which can cause lower back pain.[10]

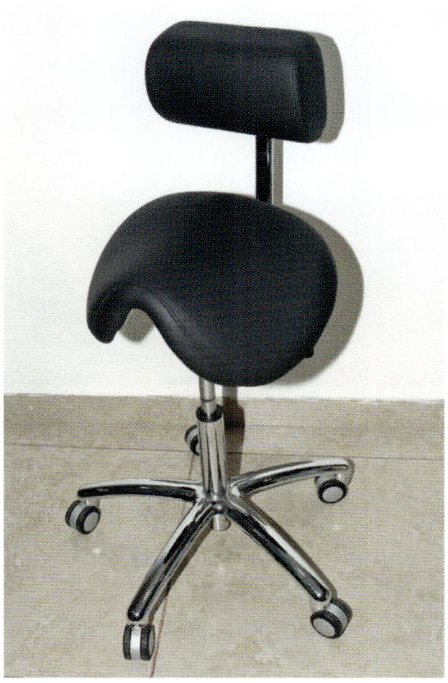

FIG 6-7 Saddle stool with backrest.

Triangular or saddle-like shape seat pans are also available on the market with the same concept, opening the hip angle and preserving the natural lumbar curve. These stool models allow closer proximity to the patient by opening the angle of the hips, which places the body in the most neutral sitting posture[11] (Fig 6-7).

Backrest

A good backrest with good lumbar support maintains the spinal curve in seated posture.[6] The lumbar support is the convex portion on which the curve of the lower back rests. The backrest must be approximately 20 cm tall to provide adequate support of the concave lumbar curve. In the case of longer lumbar supports, it must be evaluated whether the support promotes an adequate convexity of the lumbar curve and does not press forward on the thoracic curve where support is not necessary. Lumbar support should allow an up-and-down adjustment to suit the operator's height in the curve of the lumbar spine[2] (see Fig 6-4).

There are smart stool designs that allow frequent or dynamic movement of the spine that could be beneficial in reducing lower back pain.[12] The dynamic movement of the backrest of some stool brands while sitting may produce a healthy environment for blood flow through the muscles. This will allow an open nutrient pathway, which means more oxygen in the tissues, contraction and relaxing of muscles, and removal of metabolic waste products (healthy physiologic environment). In this way, not only will lower back pain and muscle activity be reduced in the stabilizer muscles, but the working posture will also be improved. This design promotes active sitting, but it does not limit the pelvis to a single position, as with a flat seat.

This innovation allows for spine and pelvis movement because the chair adapts to the body and not the other way around. When trying the stool, a good back support design will put pressure on the back where necessary, in the fulcrum lumbar area, not higher on the thoracic spine. It will also put the discs in the best physiologic situation.[13]

The shape of the backrest is extremely important for the purpose of lower back support. The first chairs that I acquired had very wide and concave backrests in the lumbar area, leaving a void in this area where there was no muscle contact. The idea of a convex lumbar support that can be adjusted directly in the lumbar area could be effective to provide true support in this highly overused area. Remember, this is the area where the fulcrum points are generated and where the postural muscles of the back are located. These muscles work hard to keep the rest of the trunk in an upright position.[14,15] It has also been found that, when sitting against the backrest, muscle activity in the postural muscles of the back and the abdominal obliques decreases.[16]

Proper adjustment of the backrest height and pressure against the lumbar lordosis is ideal to provide the support where needed and to avoid excessive pressure of the backrest pushing forward, making the operator slide in the seat. If it is not possible to purchase an ergonomic stool and the current stool is not as well designed, it can be adjusted with an air-filled wedge-shaped cushion for better back support. This is an engineering control that can be applied to the existing workspace.[2]

Armrest

The main characteristic of the armrest is its ability to adjust to provide the operator with upper limb support in balanced neutral posture. On average, the arms make up 5.33% of total body weight.[17] We know that this weight in static postures and in frequent movements outside the neutral posture results in stress and fatigue in the shoulder, elbow, and wrist joints. Added to the force of gravity, this places the upper limbs at risk for the development of musculoskeletal disorders. Shoulder muscle activity has been shown to increase with abduction and flexion angles. As the shoulder angles increase by separating the arm from the midpoint of the body, muscular pressure increases in the muscles that produce the motion or posture when passing 30 degrees of arm abduction.[18]

Studies report that the use of armrests helps prevent pain in the neck, shoulder, and back,[19] especially preventing overworking of the musculature, obstruction of the blood nutrition pathway, and creation of pressure in the joints and muscles produced by isometric contractions to be able to maintain the posture.[20] There is also some evidence of low levels of upper trapezius muscle activation with the use of arm supports when compared with no arm supports. If properly adjusted and used, arm supports can distribute the forces and weight of the arms.[21,22]

The support of the hands and arms provided by the armrest also allows for improved micromotor skills required for dentistry and surgery, improving not only the operator's comfort but also their performance of the surgical task.[23,24] The use of the armrest in dentistry, by supporting either the elbow or forearm, generates that support to execute movements with both hands: the hand holding the mirror and the hand actively working.

There are several types of armrests, including the adjustable fixed armrest and the movable telescopic armrest. The adjustable fixed armrest should promote adjustment of movement horizontally and vertically. The telescopic movable armrest provides the operator a wide range of movements of the arm support, laterally and anteroposteriorly. This helps to execute movements of horizontal distance, such as taking the handpiece and repositioning it in the side delivery system, picking up instruments from a tray, and exchanging instruments with the assistant. The comfort and support is always guaranteed; it is like one more extension of the operator's arms. Many general dentists using a stool with telescopic orientation armrests feel uncomfortable with their mobility spectrum and worry that they may hit the patient's head. The use of these armrests requires a prior adaptation and learning curve to take advantage of the benefits of its support at all times.

The operator can lean on the armrest with the elbow or the forearm, depending on the task to be carried out; both are efficient fulcrum points to work with if supported by the armrest. However, the material it is made of plays a role in the comfort of its use (eg, cushioned/padded or not).

Adjusting the height is essential to avoid neck and shoulder discomfort and pain. Setting it too low or too high may increase pressure in these areas. If located too high, it could compromise the operator's posture by forcing them to lean forward or to chronically abduct their arms.[25] Adjusting the width of the armrests is also very important; this distance is measured with hip breadth sitting, approximately 18 inches. Therefore, it is fundamental to adjust the armrest according to each operator, considering the size of the limbs and the body, because each body adjusts to the support that we attach to the chair. The height of the armrests should match the level of the elbows when relaxed.

TABLE 6-1 Cylinder sizes and heights in most stool brands on the market

Cylinder size	Lowest position (inches)	Highest position (inches)
Small	18.5	22.2
Medium	20	24–25
Standard	21	27.75
Large	22.25	30.25
X-large	26.25	36

Height

One of the main considerations in stool selection is the height of the stool, measured with the stool cylinder. The height of the cylinder should be customized to the operator based on their anthropometric measurements. Cylinder height can directly impact musculoskeletal health in seated work posture. Some chairs come with a standard cylinder height and do not allow adjustment for every operator. Ideally, however, an ergonomic stool should provide adjustability and height selection. Many stools and cylinders available on the market have several heights, varying from 18.5 to 25 inches, and even longer heights are available for taller operators[26] (Table 6-1).

Foot ring of assistant's stool

The foot ring can be adjusted to any height and will give extra support for the legs. This is very useful for short assistants because the seat may need to be high for the assistant to view the patient's mouth.

Patient Chair

One of the most frequent mistakes in purchasing the patient chair is considering the comfort of the patient over the comfort of the operator, assistant, and hygienist. The comfort of the dental staff should come first, and the patient's comfort should come second. For example, a wide backrest may make it more difficult for the operator or assistant to reach the oral cavity, requiring them to bend further and putting additional strain on their back and muscles.[2] There are several brands of patient chairs on the market, with various features (eg, with or without spittoon), sizes, shapes, and materials.

Some practices use the so-called *Beach concept*, a working table designed by Daryl Beach, rather than a classic dental chair. This method has been practiced in Japan since the 1950s and seems to promote a better posture for the operator.[27] With this method, the dentist is mainly seated at 12 o'clock and uses a mirror for an indirect view of the oral cavity. Four-handed dentistry is practiced with the assistant providing water, suction, and cleaning of the mirror. The table provides versatile patient positioning with a side delivery system for easy reach of handpieces and other instruments in the correct direction. A patient headrest is also included with wrist supports for the operator and favorable leverage near the patient's mouth.

The dental chair and delivery system selection are critical decision factors when starting from scratch with the office design. These elements must benefit the posture and workflow of the clinician and staff. Essential considerations are the size of the operatory and the number of people who will be using the space—there must be enough room for everyone to move around even when all the furniture is in place.

There must be enough room for everyone to move around even when all the furniture is in place.

When selecting a patient chair, the following factors should be considered:

- Accessibility to the patient by the assistant and operator
- Gaining visual access for the operator
- Mobility within the operatory
- Comfort for the patient

Headrest

An important consideration in the design of the patient chair is the headrest. A wide headrest can make it more difficult for the dentist and assistant to reach the patient's oral cavity, taking them out of neutral posture. It may also get in the way of the operator's legs, obstructing them from moving close enough to the patient. For these reasons, a patient chair with a small, slim headrest is recommended.

Dual-articulated and magnetic headrests may allow great flexibility in terms of patient positioning. This allows the patient's head to be moved in strategic positions to allow the operator the best view of certain tooth surfaces. Some dentists who use the optical microscope remove the headrest of the chair and instead place a foam pillow for the cervical support of the patient's head. This allows the operator to get even closer to the oral cavity while providing comfort to the patient at the same time.

Backrest

Like the headrest, the backrest should be slim and narrow. This allows for the best proximity and accessibility for the dentist to move around, see what they need to see, and reach where they need to reach. The market has a variety of styles for patient chair backrests, and those with wings or additional width can obstruct the ideal position to access the patient's mouth, particularly in the 9 o'clock to 12 o'clock positions.[28] Not only does this promote leaning and bending forward from the trunk, but it also obstructs the proper workflow between the assistant, patient, and operator.

Height

The height of the patient chair must be adjustable to allow the operator to achieve a neutral posture. When the height reach of the chair is not enough and does not allow the patient to be lifted, it may not be possible to obtain an adequate working distance to the patient. If the patient is too low in the chair, the operator is forced to lean into the patient's mouth in order to get adequate vision or lower the microscope accordingly, thereby requiring the head-down nonneutral posture over 20 degrees.

Armrest

Most patient chairs comes with two fixable sling-style armrests that provide patient support while lying on the chair. These can be adjusted laterally outward or removed to allow comfortable entry and exit of the patient to and from the chair.

Swivel feature

If there is minimal space between the patient chair and other office furniture, having a swivel feature can be helpful to move around, turn, and gain access to the patient's head.[2]

Length

Most chairs on the market range from 70 to 75 inches in length with the headrest fully extended. The most important consideration is that the office dimensions allow a minimum of 20 inches between the edge of the head (when fully reclined) and the office furniture, so that the operator can easily move into the 12 o'clock position. This is the most recommended position to use, especially when practicing with an optical microscope.

Spittoons

Although many ergonomic chairs come with spittoons, they may be oversized and interfere with the position of the assistant. The assistant is generally between 1 o'clock and 3 o'clock, around the same location as the spittoon. We recommend choosing a patient chair that does not include a spittoon; it saves space and allows appropriate accommodation and mobility for the assistant.

Orientation of patient chair

The orientation of the patient chair in the office can greatly affect the posture and body mechanics of the operator. It is vital that there be a space of at least 20 inches behind the patient's head to allow the operator work in the 12 o'clock position; working at this location allows for the most neutral working posture. If this is not

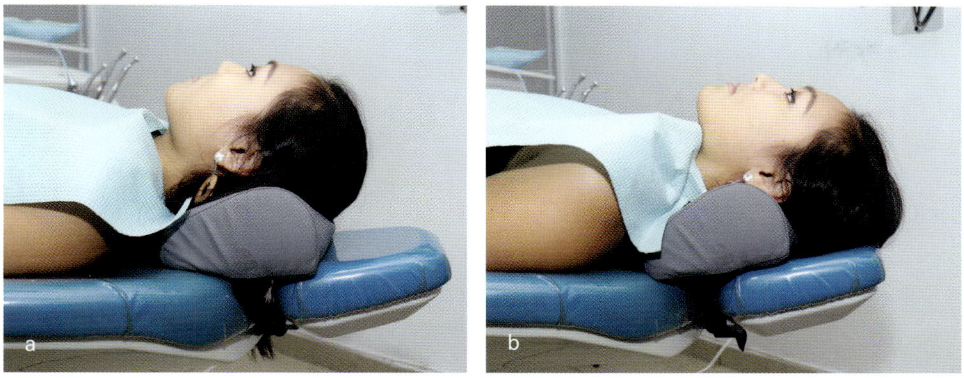

FIG 6-8 *(a)* The patient's head is too far forward for the operator to reach. *(b)* Ideal position for the patient with their head at the very end of the headrest.

possible, try to rotate the patient chair 15 to 20 degrees to gain access to the 12 o'clock position. Strategic positioning is everything in dentistry.

Strategic positioning is everything in dentistry.

It should be remembered that the patient chair is not usually stationary in the office and can be moved a few centimeters, depending on where your electrical box is located. Modifying the chair closer or further from the counter or at a different angle can improve the ergonomics of the entire work team.

Position of patient in chair

The main objective in the positioning of the patient is to promote the operator's comfort. The patient is in the dental chair a limited time, and the operator sits in a similar position every day throughout their career. It is key to communicate your needs verbally to the patient, directing them to the position most convenient for you. Depending on the quadrant to work on, you can ask the patient to turn the head to one side or the other for better visual access. Instruct the patient to place their head at the end of the headrest. Leaving a space between the end of the headrest and the operator would move the patient's oral cavity away from the operator, requiring them to tilt forward (Fig 6-8). The biomechanical risks of this motion, discussed in previous chapters, can be avoided with a simple verbal instruction.

There are some special comfortable neck cushions for the patient that are usually of great help (see Fig 6-8). At the same time, they allow for gain of a few centimeters of focal length when we work with the microscope. A neck cushion can also be helpful if the patient is small or if the chair cannot be raised high enough for operator comfort.

The ideal height for the patient is one in which the occlusal surfaces of the teeth to be worked on are at the level of the operator's elbow or slightly

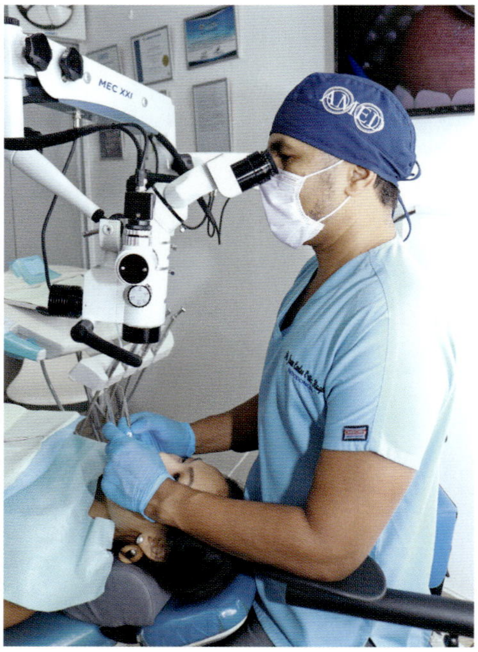

FIG 6-9 Ideal position of the operator's elbows in relation to the patient's mouth.

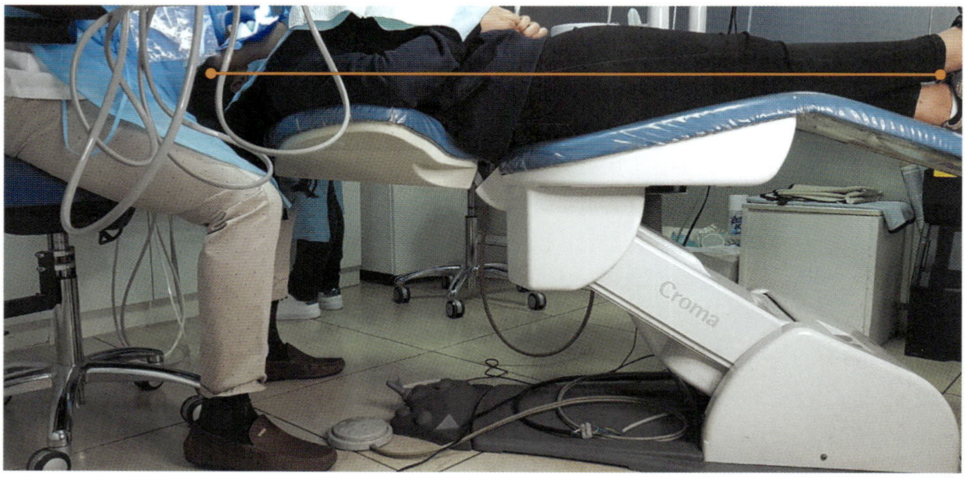

FIG 6-10 Ideal horizontal position of the patient in the chair.

higher[11] (Fig 6-9). This will ensure that the working surface (the mouth of the patient) is in the operator's seated power zone for the least stress and fatigue on the body. The dentist's forearms and wrist will tend to be near or in the neutral posture zone. In microscope dentistry, the mouth of the patient determines the height of the microscope position, and the height of the microscope sets the position of the operator's head. Remember, the operator's head should sit straight with the ears above the shoulders with no inclination of the neck.

It is recommended to place the dental chair as horizontally as possible so that all quadrants in the mouth can be reached strategically without visual obstructions, facilitating easy work on all tooth surfaces (Fig 6-10). When working with a microscope, tilting the patient chair will alter the focal length of the microscope

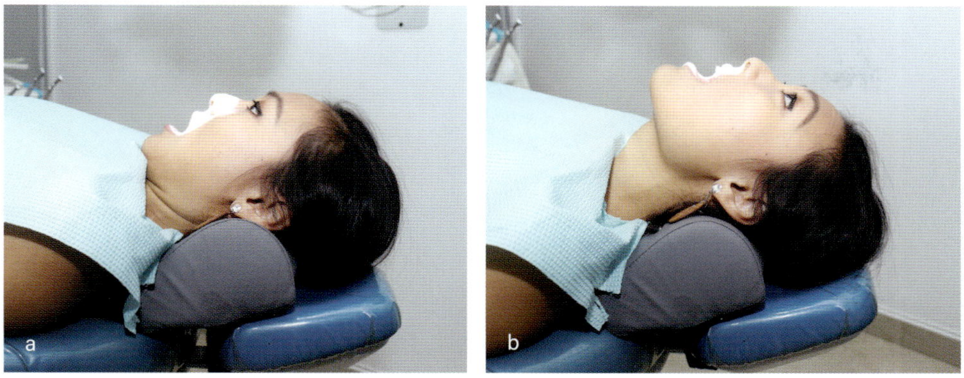

FIG 6-11 *(a)* Position of the patient's chin toward the chest. *(b)* Position of the chin up. Verbal cues instructing the patient on positioning allow better visualization of different tooth surfaces.

as the mouth is brought closer. This will then require the head of the microscope to be raised, modifying the position of the eyepieces at 90 degrees and causing an overstretch or hyperextension of the operator's head. If the backrest is partly tilted, the patient's cheeks and nose may obstruct direct view of some surfaces, in turn generating nonneutral postures in the operator's back, neck, and wrists.

A generally horizontal position of the chair backrest can keep a consistent position of the head of the microscope and therefore the focal length. In this way, the position of the operator's head does not need to be altered and can remain in neutral posture, creating a healthy environment for musculoskeletal tissues. Depending on which teeth and which arch are being worked on, the patient can be instructed to move their chin toward their chest or raise it toward the ceiling (Fig 6-11). This is done to create a more direct line of visual access for the operator.[29]

In conjunction with verbal instructions, the dentist may also turn the patient's head laterally by placing their hands on the patient's zygomatic area. This can be done when visual access to specific areas is needed and more convenient than leaving neutral posture or moving the microscope. By communicating with the patient, we can gain working comfort and therefore improve clinical results.

Patient positioning should be performed in the following sequence:

1. Incline the dental chair horizontally.
2. Move the patient's head to the end of the headrest.
3. Adjust the dental chair to the appropriate height.
4. Instruct the patient to move their head and chin in the directions you need to access the appropriate quadrant and tooth surfaces.

Delivery Systems

There are different delivery systems available on the market: rear, side, and over the patient. When a system is being purchased, the salesperson may focus primarily on esthetics or productivity. However, you should first consider the space that

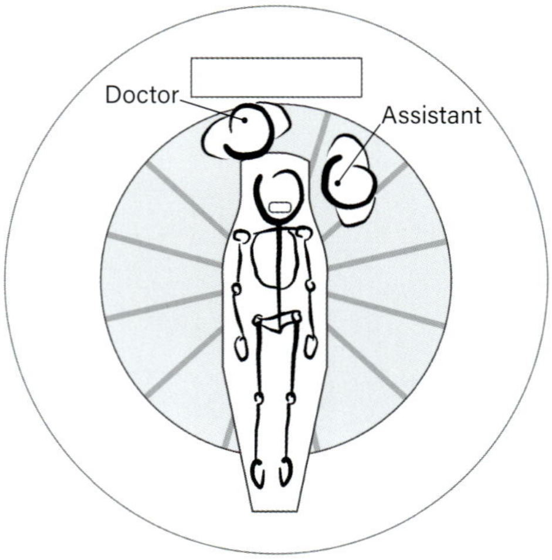

FIG 6-12 Rear delivery system. Ergonomically, this is the best system when working with an assistant (four-handed dentistry).

exists in the office and the advantages and disadvantages of different delivery systems based on this space. Having this understanding will help you select the equipment that is most appropriate for your individual office and work team.[30]

It is important to consider the positions of the operator and assistant during active work. This will depend on factors like the available space in the office, the position of cabinets, the delivery system, the type of dental chair, whether a microscope is used, and more. Having these aspects arranged in a manner that allows fluid movement will lead to an ergonomic work practice.

Rear delivery systems

This type of system positions the instruments behind the operator, which allows larger equipment to be placed in front of the operator (Fig 6-12). In my personal opinion, this system is the best ergonomically. One of its main advantages is that it allows four-handed dentistry by having the handpieces, triple syringe, suction, tray, and other instruments at the fingertips of the assistant and operator, ensuring an ideal workflow and horizontal reaching for both of them, promoting good motion economics.[31] The constant-use instruments will be in front of the assistant, allowing a reaching proximity to transfer the instruments to the operator. Another advantage is that there should be enough space on either side of the patient chair for the operator and assistant to move around without difficulty. In addition, because the patient cannot see the instruments, it may reduce anxiety in patients who are apprehensive about treatment.

The rear delivery system is the worst type of system to implement if the dentist is working without an assistant.

However, the rear delivery system is the worst type of system to implement if the dentist is working without an assistant. The dentist is obligated to rotate their body to grip instruments, abducting the upper limbs frequently throughout the day, which is a risk factor for developing pain in the lower back and shoulders.[32] If the office is arranged in this way, the operator should transfer the instruments from the nondominant to the dominant hand to avoid repetitive movements of rotation, tilt, and overreaching.[33] Therefore, if the office is designed to work without an assistant (two-handed dentistry), it would be advisable to use another system.

Some rear delivery systems do not allow proper movement in the 12 o'clock position (the healthiest, ergonomically speaking). This forces the operator to move to work positions closer to 10 o'clock or 11 o'clock if there is not enough space between the end of the patient's headrest and the rear delivery system.

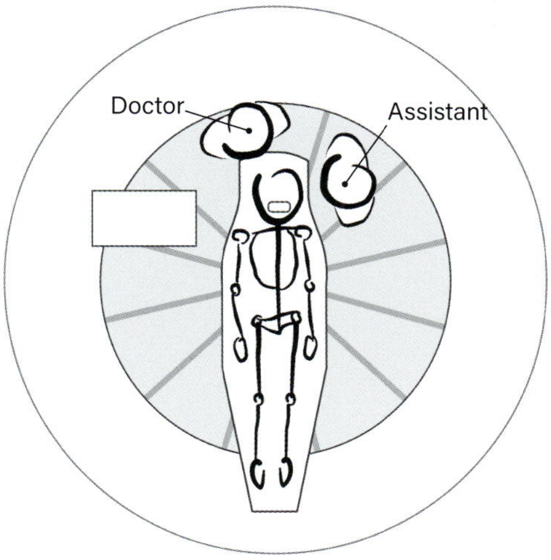

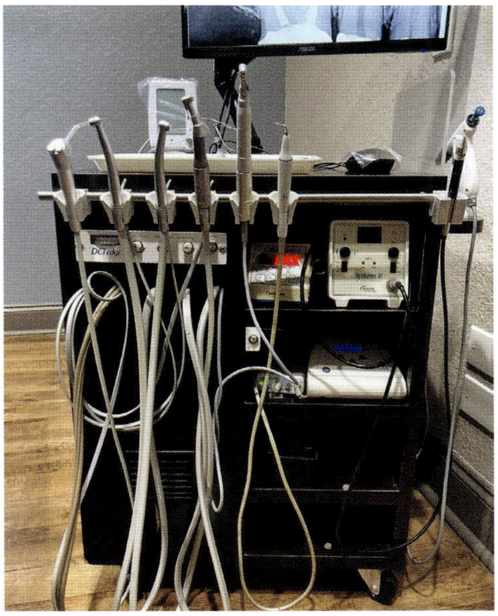

FIG 6-13 *(left)* Side delivery system. The dentist can easily access the system, but the assistant cannot.

FIG 6-14 *(right)* Example of movable side delivery system. This is generally used in endodontics to work with all the adapted handpieces and instruments together with software and a monitor to manage all instruments in one unit.

Side delivery systems

The idea behind a side delivery system is a smooth workflow throughout the procedure with the fewest interruptions (Fig 6-13). When placed properly, this type of system requires less rotation of the trunk of the operator than the rear delivery system; however, it limits the assistant's ability to reach the instruments on the tray. As a result, the operator may be the one reaching for the frequent-use high-speed handpiece, low-speed handpiece, and triple syringe. This can cause the operator to maintain a single position hour after hour, day after day, which causes overwork, fatigue, and consequently pain.[33] As discussed in chapter 2, dynamic movement is essential to maintain spine and muscle health.

To facilitate dynamic movement, the side delivery system can be modified by a movable cart (Fig 6-14). Most moveable carts on the market have triple syringe, light-curing lamps, high-speed and low-speed handpieces, and other specialized instruments. Using a mobile delivery system allows the instruments to be in close proximity to the operator or the assistant as needed. It is a good idea to locate the side delivery system near the operator's hands, placing the handpieces and triple syringe at a comfortable reaching distance. The operator's arm should still be supported by the armrest when picking equipment up, and it should be easy to replace instruments in the assistant's hands, other trays, or the mobiliary.

Some setups have equipment such as lasers or CAD/CAM equipment next to and in front of the operator, and a side delivery system may interfere with positioning of this equipment. There are also cabinetry systems available with adjustable mounted side delivery systems. These are foldable and extendable to be placed under the worktop when not in use and can be adjusted to the most convenient height and distance for the operator.

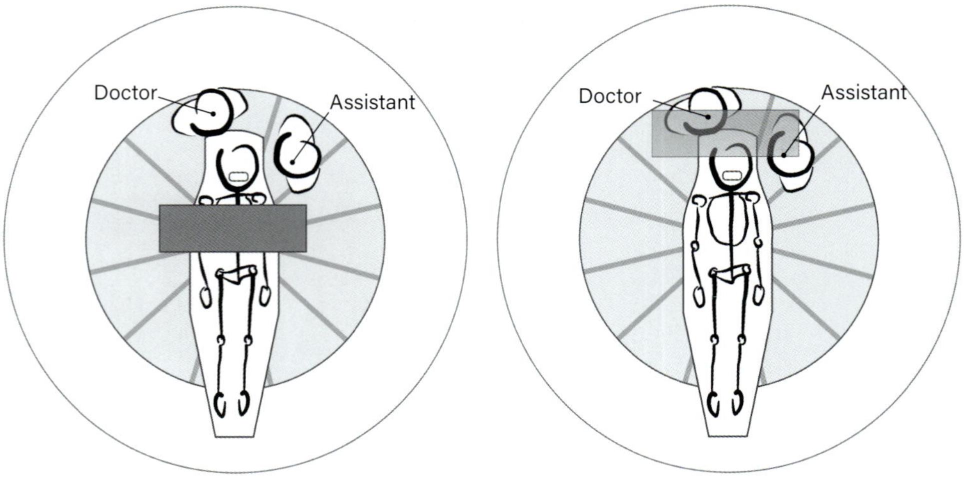

FIG 6-15 *(left)* Delivery system over the patient's chest.

FIG 6-16 *(right)* Delivery system over the patient's head.

Over-the-patient delivery systems

This system allows free movement around the patient's head in the positions from 9 o'clock to 12 o'clock. The unit is placed above the patient's chest; in this way, handpieces and other instruments are within easy reach for both the operator and the assistant (Fig 6-15). However, this system is close to the patient and can be a problem if the patient is very large. This system is ideal for four-handed dentistry and still acceptable for two-handed dentistry due to the proximity of the tray, handpieces, suction, and triple syringe.

Another type of over-the-patient delivery system is one that is over the patient's head rather than their chest (Fig 6-16). This type of delivery system is one of the newest on the market, and it has similar benefits and disadvantages as the rear delivery system. It is being recognized as one of the best delivery systems because it combines the benefits of the rear delivery system and the over-the-chest delivery system.[31] It also allows the operator to work in the widest range of positions around the head of the patient. The supplies are in an ideal position for the assistant, while the handpieces are more accessible than in the rear delivery system, which reduces the challenges of two-handed dentistry.

Office Layout and Design

The office layout and design should be governed by the idea of comfort, health, and productivity of the operator and work staff. When it comes to remodeling or designing an office from scratch, important factors must be taken into account, such as necessary space, smart furniture design, and areas of the office that allow fluid four-handed work. Workplace design is critical to attain efficiency and productivity within the job. Ergonomically oriented workspace design promotes efficient workflow and the most favorable environment for proper posture and positioning for the dental team systematically and sequentially.[34]

A good workstation layout should be oriented mainly by respecting horizontal reaching distances for constant-use, frequent-use, and occasional-use instruments and equipment. As a team, the operator, hygienist, assistant, and office staff should know what items are used during treatment. Those items can then be prepared between patients in sequential order, and patients can be positioned on the chair considering reaching distance to the patient's mouth.[35]

Some of these factors directly affect the posture and body mechanics of the operator and assistant. It is recommended to enlist a professional industrial designer or architect to appropriately plan the space. Decisions made at this stage will impact the health of the staff members and the long-term success of the practice.

The primary objective of office design is easy reach of equipment, supplies, and instruments by the operator and the assistant. When your office is small, accommodating all the products is a challenge, and ideally they should be located at your fingertips.[36] A helpful starting point is to consider the dimensions and size of the operatory when choosing the furniture and delivery system.

The primary objective of office design is easy reach of equipment, supplies, and instruments by the operator and the assistant.

Equipment used only occasionally should be placed farther away or on a cart that can be moved between offices. The ideal location of equipment can be determined by moving your forearms in a horizontal arc with your elbows relaxed on the sides of the body. This creates a radius of approximately 15.7 inches for both the dentist and the assistant, and all constant-use equipment should be within this radius. Frequent-use equipment can have a wider radius of about 21.9 inches from the shoulder when the elbow is extended. This equipment is mainly handled by the assistant rather than the dentist. Consolidating these primary work areas can increase productivity and decrease unnecessary movements while promoting the comfort and musculoskeletal health of the assistant and operator.

A good concept is placing the delivery system, primary instruments, and handpieces away from the hand but within minimum reach of the operator and assistant. If these elements are placed out of range, the operator and assistant will have to perform repetitive overreaching movements to access them, increasing the risk of developing musculoskeletal disorders in the lower back, arms, shoulder, and neck (Fig 6-17).

Counter and delivery system height

To prevent neck and shoulder dysfunction, the counter, delivery system, and the patient's oral cavity must at the same height as the operator's elbows when sitting with arms relaxed to the sides.[37] As mentioned previously, the dimensions of the room will be the determinants for the best choice of furniture, including counters. Whether a new office is being designed or an existing office is being modified, a professional designer should be consulted and should consider the operator's body measurements in their design. Counters are frequently manufactured at a standard height, which can create ergonomic problems when the user does not fit that standard. For example, tall operators must lean forward and down to pick up instruments on counters 80 centimeters high (standard measure). The best

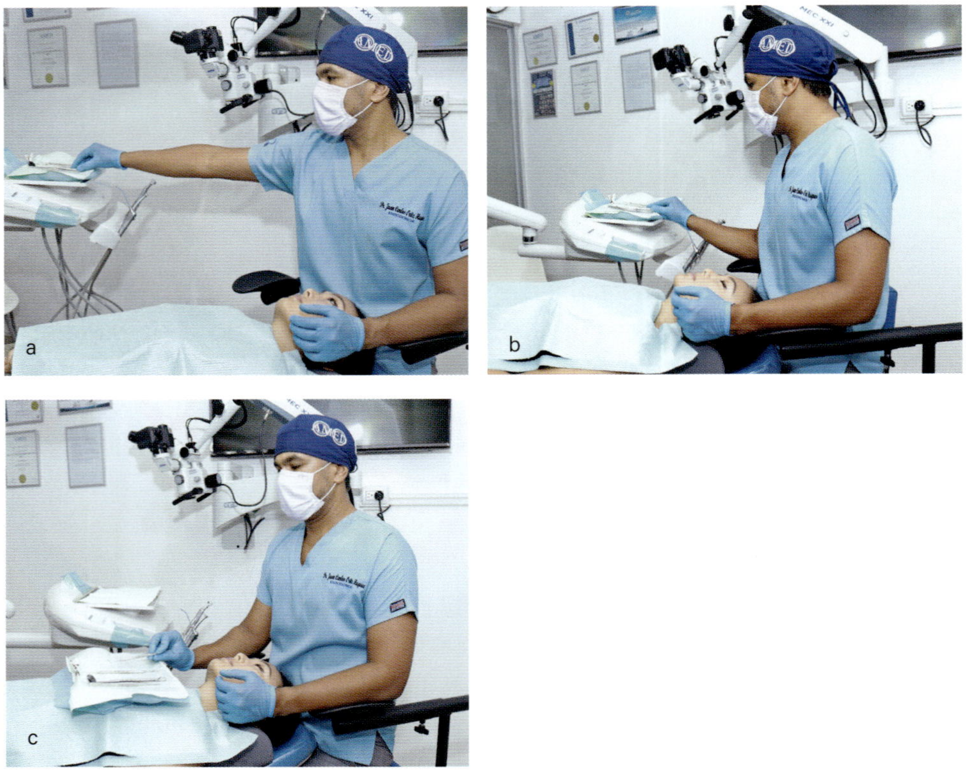

FIG 6-17 *(a)* The tray is placed too far away, and abduction and arm extension from the shoulder are required to reach the instruments. *(b)* This delivery system allows instruments to be reached with minimal abduction and arm extension, with the operator remaining in the neutral position. *(c)* Ideal position with instruments at minimum reach distances.

way to solve this type of problem is to reduce the reach distance to supplies. For tall operators, it may be better to use wall cabinets that do not extend to the floor.

The dental cabinet that stores supplies and instruments of frequent or constant use should ideally be installed in a location where the operator and the assistant can reach instruments and materials with equal ease. These instruments can be prepared in advance depending on the schedule and type of procedure to be performed. This way, trays with instruments can be ready before the patient gets into the operatory, saving time, reducing the need to rush, and resulting in less fatigue.

Assistant delivery systems

Using mobile carts or cabinetry can solve the frequent problem of excessive movements required by the assistant to reach instruments. This often occurs in instances of classic fixed furniture that is too far from the dental chair. The main problem with wall systems is that they frequently force the assistant to leave their position to go looking for supplies. This interrupts the work, which may also create mental fatigue.

The most ergonomic assistant delivery system is one that is mobile. These systems provide a versatile operatory layout that can be adjusted to any dental procedure, patient, dentist, and assistant, enhancing time and workflow efficiency[2] (Fig 6-18). A mobile cart can have multiple drawers for storage and can be purchased premade or custom-designed for your office depending on the available space and preferred positioning.

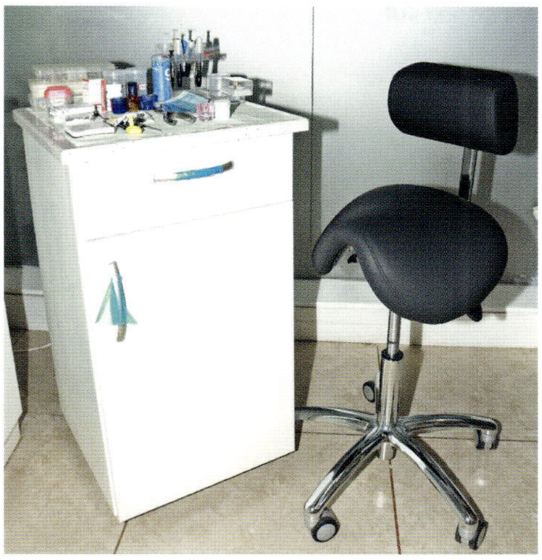

FIG 6-18 Movable assistant cart.

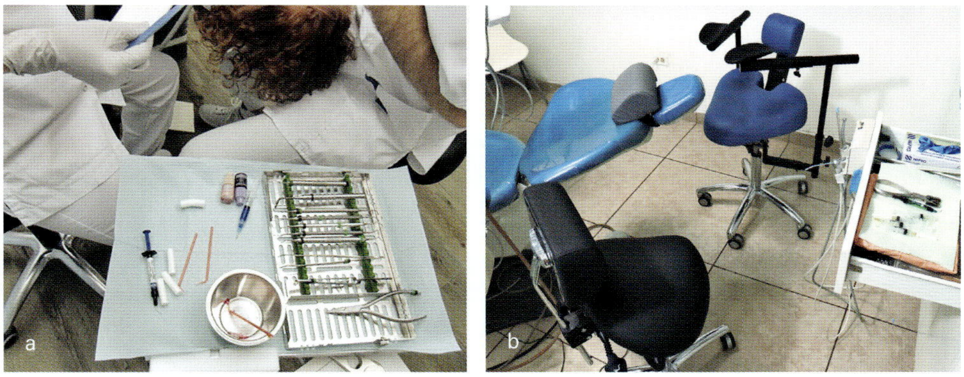

FIG 6-19 *(a and b)* Existing cabinetry can be modified or used differently to keep the delivery system behind the patient but extend the instruments closer to the operator and assistant.

Another option is to modify cabinetry behind the patient. Trays can be added with special hinges that allow them to be extended to the hands of the assistant and the operator (Fig 6-19). When working with an existing office layout that cannot be redesigned, look for ways to modify the space or purchase new equipment to make the workflow easier and more comfortable for the operator and the assistant.

Utilities

Suction and triple syringe are probably the two most important delivery system utilities. Because these two utilities are constantly used by the assistant, they have to be in easy reach and in the assistant's line of view so trunk rotation is not required to access them. On some occasions, the suction is close to the spittoon and is behind the assistant, requiring the assistant to rotate to be able to take the suction. Some chairs only have the triple syringe on the dentist's side, which can be a problem in side delivery systems because both constant-use items are out of reach of the assistant. These are examples of poor ergonomic design in the dental chair manufacturing industries, as this dental chair setting can influence the working dynamics within the operatory.

Suction and triple syringe are probably the two most important delivery system utilities.

Some systems include an extendable arm for the utilities, allowing them to be placed in front of the assistant even if the system itself is further away. As mentioned previously, mobile systems are also useful in this regard. It can be very helpful to have an adjustable tray that allows suction and triple syringe to be close to the assistant and dentist when needed but out of the way when not needed. Adding this functionality is an ergonomic engineering modification that can help when the delivery system in your office is already set.

Machinery and dental technology

Technology has become essential in dental offices today. This type of equipment includes computers, monitors, digital x-ray sensors, and more. The main computer should be placed out of the line of sight for dental procedures, preferably behind the operator or assistant at the 12 o'clock or 2 o'clock position. It is used for storing and accessing digital data on the patient, x-ray sensor software, videos from the optical microscope, and files related to patient treatment.[38] Different systems can be used such as an all-in-one system or a laptop or computer with an external hard drive. The best system to use will depend on the design and counter space available. Less is more; counters should be kept as clean and clear as possible to avoid clutter or cramping things into a space that is too small.

The computer keyboard must be located at a height that allows the operator's forearms to be parallel to the floor or tilted slightly upward. This is difficult to accomplish with a laptop because the keyboard and monitor are at the same height. The mouse space should also be considered. A wireless mouse and keyboard are preferred because there are fewer limitations with regard to their positioning, allowing for smoother movements. The top of the computer monitor should be at the same level as the operator's eyes to place the head in the most neutral posture.[39]

The location of the monitor is of utmost importance from an ergonomic perspective. Ideally, there should be two monitors in the dentist's office: one located behind and at the right side of the operator in the line of view of the assistant, and another facing or above the patient[40] (Fig 6-20). One way or another, monitors should generally be in close range, and the top of the monitor should be slightly below the patient's eye level.

The patient/dentist monitor can be used to display photographs, live videos, and radiographs, improving communication between the dentist and patient as well as helping the patient to understand the diagnoses and treatments. The position most convenient for live images while the operator works would be one mounted from the ceiling (see Fig 6-20), because it allows the patient to observe them comfortably while lying down.[40] The monitor size will depend on the proximity to the patient. If you are at a considerable distance, a larger screen is recommended. There is a visual rule stating that a double distance of the screen would take four times the screen size to get the same detail. In other words, a 15-inch monitor at 60 centimeters is equivalent to a 30-inch monitor at 120 centimeters.

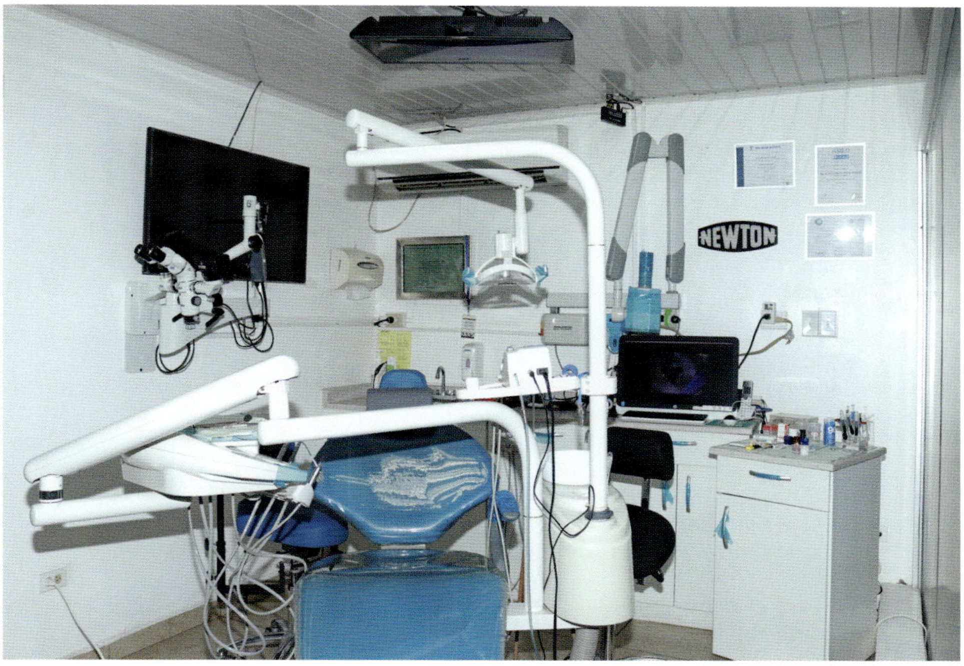

FIG 6-20 Monitors placed in different positions in the office.

Conclusion

Remember that *how* you use something matters more than what you use. Whether musculoskeletal problems will develop depends not on the acquisition of ergonomically designed equipment but on the adjustments and proper use of the equipment you have. Equipment should be fitted to the person using it, customized or adjusted to their body. Patient chairs should be designed and selected with the operator's comfort in mind more so than the patient's; they should be small enough for the operator and assistant to comfortably move around as necessary and get as close as possible to the patient's head. Using a specially designed table instead of a chair for the patient may be of benefit as well. The delivery system and cabinetry of choice will depend on the size of the operatory and the preference of operator and assistant position around the patient.

References

1. Rising DW, Bennett BC, Hursh K, Plesh O. Reports of body pain in a dental student population. J Am Dent Assoc 2005;136:81–86.
2. Valachi B. Practice Dentistry Pain-Free: Evidence-Based Strategies to Prevent Pain and Extend Your Career. Portland, OR: Posturedontics, 2008.
3. Finkbeiner BL. Are you ready to switch to four-handed dentistry? Dentistry IQ. https://www.dentistryiq.com/practice-management/staffing/article/16348394/are-you-ready-to-switch-to-fourhanded-dentistry. Accessed 24 March 2022.
4. Rundcrantz BL, Johnsson B, Moritz U. Cervical pain and discomfort among dentists. Epidemiological, clinical and therapeutic aspects. Part 1. A survey of pain and discomfort. Swed Dent J 1990;14:71–80.
5. Harrison DD, Harrison SO, Croft AC, Harrison DE, Troyanovich SJ. Sitting biomechanics part I: Review of the literature. J Manipulative Physiol Ther 1999;22:594–609.
6. Snijders CJ, Hermans PF, Niesing R, Spoor CW, Stoeckart R. The influence of slouching and lumbar support on iliolumbar ligaments, intervertebral discs and sacroiliac joints. Clin Biomech (Bristol, Avon) 2004;19:323–329.

7. Anderson LM, Helander MG. The effects of spinal shrinkage and comfort of a forwardly-inclined seat with and without a backrest. Proceedings of the International Ergonomics Association Conference on Human Factors in Design for Manufacturability and Process Planning, 1990.
8. Valachi B. The Ergonomic Benefits of Saddle-Style Stools. Dental Products Report. https://www.dentalproductsreport.com/view/ergonomic-benefits-saddle-style-stools. Accessed 30 March 2022.
9. De Bruyne MA, Van Renterghem B, Baird A, Palmans T, Danneels L, Dolphens M. Influence of different stool types on muscle activity and lumbar posture among dentists during a simulated dental screening task. Appl Ergon 2016;56:220–226.
10. Valachi B. The Benefits of Saddle Stools in Dentistry. Posturedontics. https://posturedontics.com/saddle-up/. Accessed 30 March 2022.
11. Chaffin DB, Andersson GBJ, Martin BJ. Occupational Biomechanics, ed 4. Hoboken, NJ: John Wiley & Sons, 2006.
12. McGill S. Low Back Disorders: Evidence-Based Prevention and Rehabilitation. Champaign, IL: Human Kinetics, 2002.
13. Mandal AC, Haaksma E. Homo Sendens: The Seated Man and Back Complaints. The Hague: The Hague Clinic, Back Training & Advisory Centre.
14. Makhsous M, Lin F, Hendrix RW, Hepler M, Zhang LQ. Sitting with adjustable ischial and back supports: Biomechanical changes. Spine (Phila Pa 1976) 2003;28:1113–1122.
15. Carcone SM, Keir PJ. Effects of backrest design on biomechanics and comfort during seated work. Appl Ergon 2007;38:755–764.
16. Yoo WG. Comparison of sitting with and without a backrest during computer work. J Phys Ther Sci 2012;24:409–410.
17. Plagenhoef S, Evans FG, Abdelnour T. Anatomical data for analyzing human motion. Res Q Exerc Sport 1983;54:169–178.
18. Antony NT, Keir PJ. Effects of posture, movement and hand load on shoulder muscle activity. J Electromyogr Kinesiol 2010;20:191–198.
19. Parsell DE, Weber MD, Anderson BC, Cobb GW Jr. Evaluation of ergonomic dental stools through clinical simulation. Gen Dent 2000;48:440–444.
20. Valachi B, Valachi K. Mechanisms leading to musculoskeletal disorders in dentistry. J Am Dent Assoc 2003;134:1344–1350.
21. Bolderman FW, Bos-Huizer JJA, Hoozemans MJM. The effect of arm supports on muscle activity, posture, and discomfort in the neck and shoulder in microscopic dentistry: Results of a pilot study. IISE Trans Occup Ergon Hum Factors 2017;5:92–105.
22. Visser B, de Korte E, van der Kraan I, Kuijer P. The effect of arm and wrist supports on the load of the upper extremity during VDU work. Clin Biomech (Bristol, Avon) 2000;15(suppl 1):S34–S38.
23. Heller-Ono A. To Arm Rest...This is the Dilemma! Worksite International. https://www.worksiteinternational.com/blog/to-arm-rest-or-not-to-arm-rest. Accessed 30 March 2022.
24. Galleano R, Carter F, Brown S, Frank T, Cuschieri A. Can armrests improve comfort and task performance in laparoscopic surgery? Ann Surg 2006;243:329–333.
25. Valachi BS. Operator stools: How selection and adjustment impact your health. Dent Today 2008;27:148–151.
26. Ahearn D. The eight keys to selecting great seating for long-term health. Dent Today 2005;24:128–131.
27. Neddermeyer W. The Beach system: Physiological basis for work positions [in French]. Rev Odontostomatol (Paris) 1980;9:53–57.
28. Hokwerda O, Wouters JAJ, de Ruijter RAG, Zijlstra-Shaw S. Ergonomic Requirements for Dental Equipment: Guidelines and Recommendations for Designing, Constructing and Selecting Dental Equipment. Frankfurt, Germany: European Society of Dental Ergonomics, 2006.
29. Ellis P. Team Dentistry: Chairside Procedures and Practice Management. London: Dunitz, 1991.
30. American Dental Association. An Introduction to Ergonomics: Risk Factors, MSDs, Approaches and Interventions. https://desergo.com/wp-content/uploads/OTH-White-Paper.pdf. Accessed 7 June 2021.
31. Finkbeiner BL. Selecting equipment for the ergonomic four-handed dental practice. J Contemp Dent Pract 2001;2:4452.
32. Torén A. Muscle activity and range of motion during active trunk rotation in a sitting posture. Appl Ergon 2001;32:583–591.
33. Valachi B. Can delivery systems deliver pain? Dent Pract Rep 2006;6:60–62.
34. Ahearn DJ, Sanders MJ, Turcotte C. Ergonomic design for dental offices. Work 2010;35:495–503.
35. Pheasant S, Haslegrave CM. Bodyspace: Anthropometry, Ergonomics and the Design of Work, ed 3. Boca Raton, FL: Taylor and Francis, 2006.
36. Ahearn D. Ten Essential Elements of a Productive Treatment Room – Part 1. Dent Econ 2002. https://www.dentaleconomics.com/dental-office-design/equipment-and-furniture/article/16385922/ten-essential-elements-of-a-productive-treatment-room-part-1. Accessed 7 June 2021.
37. Kroemer KHE, Grandjean E. Fitting the Task to the Human, ed 5. Philadelphia: Taylor & Francis, 1997.
38. Ahearn D. The ergonomic conundrum for technology integration. Alpha Omegan 2006;99:110–112.
39. State of California Department of Industrial Relations. Easy Ergonomics for Desktop Computer Users. https://www.dir.ca.gov/dosh/dosh_publications/computerergo.pdf. Accessed 30 March 2022.
40. Van As GA. Digital documentation and the dental operating microscope: What you see is what you get. Int J Microdent 2009;1:30–41.

Rest, Stretching, and Fitness

7

It is important to take small breaks to move and stretch. Stretching periodically prevents physical and cognitive fatigue. Taking regular breaks and stretching during the working day can lead to a longer and healthier career.[1]

Chapter objectives

- **Understand the importance of scheduling breaks for rest or movement during the workday**
- **Know the types of programmed stretches to perform during the workday**
- **Understand the role of body fitness in strengthening postural muscles and relieving stress**

Rest

Rest is defined as periods of relief from exertion, movement, or working activities. It allows for recovery from physical and mental work. Factors such as work pace, intensity, duration, and physical and mental demands will influence how much rest is required.

Consequences of lack of rest

Studies show that musculoskeletal pain has increased since 1960 due in part to long work periods without breaks.[2] In dentistry, prolonged static postures have a negative impact on the body, which leads to fatigue and pain. Rest and stretching help to prevent muscle imbalances because they allow you to maintain a normal range of motion as well as improve flexibility.[3]

Musculoskeletal fatigue affects our ability to do our job well, so rest and breaks are an important part of our workday to prevent this fatigue. All tissue that has become fatigued due to overuse can recover with underuse if rest is applied in a timely manner. Overuse that is unchecked leads to microtears at the cellular level. Behaviors such as carelessness and inadequate recovery time will delay or prevent healing.

Central fatigue is related to the psychophysical aspect of work capacity, where a feeling of tiredness or a perception of increased exertion is present even though work is performed the same as before. This may occur with tasks with high mental intensity, which are frequent in dentistry and can include seeing anxious patients, managing tight schedules, performing difficult procedures, and using high-precision skills. Work without regular breaks is more likely to lead to central fatigue even if the muscles themselves are not fatigued.[4]

Tasks that are monotonous, boring, or not stimulating are also situations in occupational ergonomics that promote central fatigue. As dentists, we repeatedly do the same procedures over and over throughout the years—even more so if we develop one specialty exclusively. Work conditions that allow the worker control of their environment, hours, and rest periods as well as proper equipment can reduce or eliminate the onset of fatigue. Rest functions as a relief period from exertion, movement, or activity, allowing the body to recover from physical as well as mental work.

The following variables will affect the appropriate recovery time:

- Intensity of the activity
- Time between cycles
- Area of the body involved
- Duration of the task

Due to the diversity in age and fitness levels of workers, exact amounts of time to recover from work tasks have not been determined. A study on the efficacy of microbreaks during the workday found that people who regularly took breaks experienced less discomfort. Furthermore, it showed no harmful effects to productivity.[1]

Practicing unhealthy workplace habits despite knowing they contribute to health issues such as back, neck, shoulder, and wrist pain among others consciously contributes to the development of all the aforementioned painful syndromes. The incorporation of regular, programmed breaks and stretching exercises is a way to prevent and eliminate this discomfort.[5]

Systematic incorporation of breaks

Working habits and work design are key aspects to promoting healthy workplaces. Creating a healthy system within the office that really takes care of the mental and physical health, safety, and well-being of workers is a moral imperative in any job.[6]

As a dentist, it can be a challenge to incorporate rest periods into the schedule. Many fall into the habit of scheduling patients back to back or not accounting for appointments that may run long. Or, because we have a financial interest in seeing as many patients as possible, we overschedule. However, this is detrimental to our bodies, which are our greatest investment. It is truly counterproductive to sacrifice health for financial gain—if we keep our bodies healthy, performance will be optimized and our careers will benefit in the long term.

Protect your greatest investment—your body!

The following are examples of opportunities to rest or take stretching breaks:

- Chairside every 30 or 45 minutes
- Between patients
- Between taking radiographs
- Consciously during extensive procedures
- While waiting for anesthesia
- During canceled appointments

The assistant should also follow scheduled rest periods for stretching, as they suffer most of the same musculoskeletal disorders as the dentist.

There are different approaches to taking breaks for the dentist, assistant, and hygienist:

- *Spontaneous:* Stop performing the task
- *Administrative:* Built into the schedule
- *Hidden:* Decrease the intensity of the work
- *Ergo breaks:* Take 30 to 180 seconds to stretch and promote circulation

If these breaks are widely spaced out, the range of trauma could exceed the repair, which would result in tissue damage. To optimize force capacity and minimize the risk of muscle tension, short breaks should be scheduled during the workday for periods of rest and movement. This will be more beneficial than long periods of stretching, rest, and movement widely spaced out.[7]

It is also beneficial to stand up during breaks. During longer breaks or at lunchtime, take a short walk or perform other activities involving movement. The idea is to get your body in motion.

Periodic Stretching

A healthy body is flexible, strong, and well-conditioned. To achieve this, it is necessary to stretch the muscles. A 5- to 10-minute stretching routine allows blood flow and temperature deep in the muscles to be increased, improving flexibility and thereby minimizing risks.[8,9] It is recommended to stretch three to four times during the workday.

Periodic stretching has been proven to be the best way to control and prevent persistent injury. As dentists, we are tasked with sitting for hours with the patient in the chair, in prolonged static posture and awkward postures. Even if you use the best equipment, maintain postural awareness, and use perfect neutral working posture, more than half the muscles of the body are working. This is exacerbated if the work is performed without a good stool and without the optical microscope, fundamental pillars of dental ergonomics.[10]

Periodic stretching has been proven to be the best way to control and prevent persistent injury.

Advantages for the body

Sustained muscle contractions in static work positions can cause ischemia by obstructing the blood flow in the muscles.[11] The dynamic movement performed by stretching promotes a healthy contraction and relaxation of the muscles; increases the flow of blood, oxygen, and nutrients; and warms the muscles up. It also prevents and treats trigger points because it is relaxing, and trigger points can be caused by emotional stress.[12] In general, we tend to lose flexibility in the opposite direction that we execute the static posture during the day.[1] Stretching in the opposite direction will improve flexibility and prevent muscle imbalances that can cause pain and cumulative trauma disorders.

After age 30 years, the spinal discs do not receive nutrients through blood flow alone. An important way that discs receive nutrients is through movement. By alternating compression and release of pressure, the spine relaxes and absorbs nutrients.[13]

Stretching should be incorporated into the daily routine and become a professional life habit. The benefits will be more than positive in the long term—I have witnessed the results myself! At the beginning, it was challenging for me to take the time to interrupt my workflow. However, once I understood what happens to my body in static postures and the associated consequences, I started to set up my mind and created a time to stop, take a break, and do five stretching exercises. I achieved this by setting a phone alarm to go off every 40 minutes. This also provides a mental break from performing these complex cases, allowing a fresh start after each break. It may seem overwhelming and challenging, but with practice, it can become an automatic routine in our working lives.

The microbreak routine allows periods of stretching, rest, or movement. Static contraction may result in a switch to anaerobic metabolism, which increases acid formation that then decreases efficiency of energy mechanisms. This will produce ischemia, muscle spasms, reduced mobility, and pain both during work time and out of the office. Peripheral fatigue and sustained muscle contraction by awkward postures will also increase inorganic phosphate accumulation effects. This means that a more forceful effort will be required to get repetitive work done, and this is most notable with eccentric or isometric work often used in dentistry.[4]

Types of stretches to do

Ergo breaks

Stretching should be incorporated into the daily routine, which includes a series of programmed stretches or "ergo breaks" for the finger and wrist flexor, hamstring, finger and wrist extensor, lower back, and neck and shoulder (Fig 7-1). The Back School has helpful resources on taking ergo breaks.[14]

Regular stretches every 30 to 45 minutes, held for 10–15 seconds, for two or three breath cycles, will promote dynamic blood flow into the tissues and muscles. Note: It is recommended to consult a health professional before starting this ergo break series if you have any health issues.

The duration of the stretches performed during microbreaks is important. Sustained stretches of 15 to 30 seconds have been shown to be more effective than repeated stretches of only 5 seconds.[15] The recommendation is to do as many stretching cycles as possible for at least 15 seconds each, every 30 to 45 minutes.[16] Imagine yourself as an athlete. Athletes use the best equipment, the best techniques, and the best body mechanics to perform at the highest level, so the dentist and staff should do the same to obtain the best results while simultaneously keeping their bodies healthy.

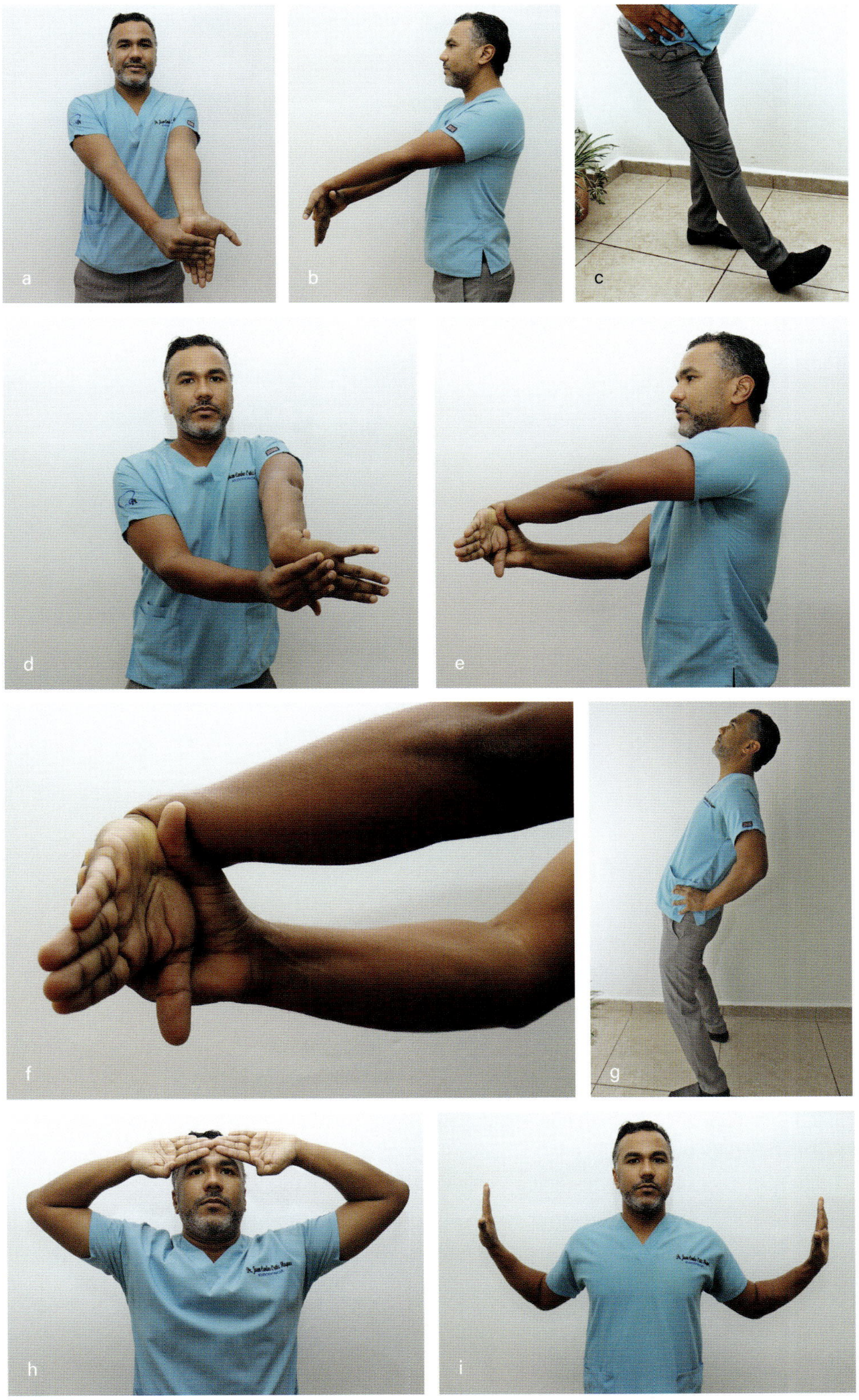

FIG 7-1 The "ergo break." *(a and b)* Finger and wrist flexor stretch. *(c)* Hamstring stretch. *(d to f)* Finger and wrist extensor stretch. *(g)* Lower back flexor stretch. *(h and i)* Neck shoulder stretch.

FIG 7-2 *(a and b)* Seated postural exercise.

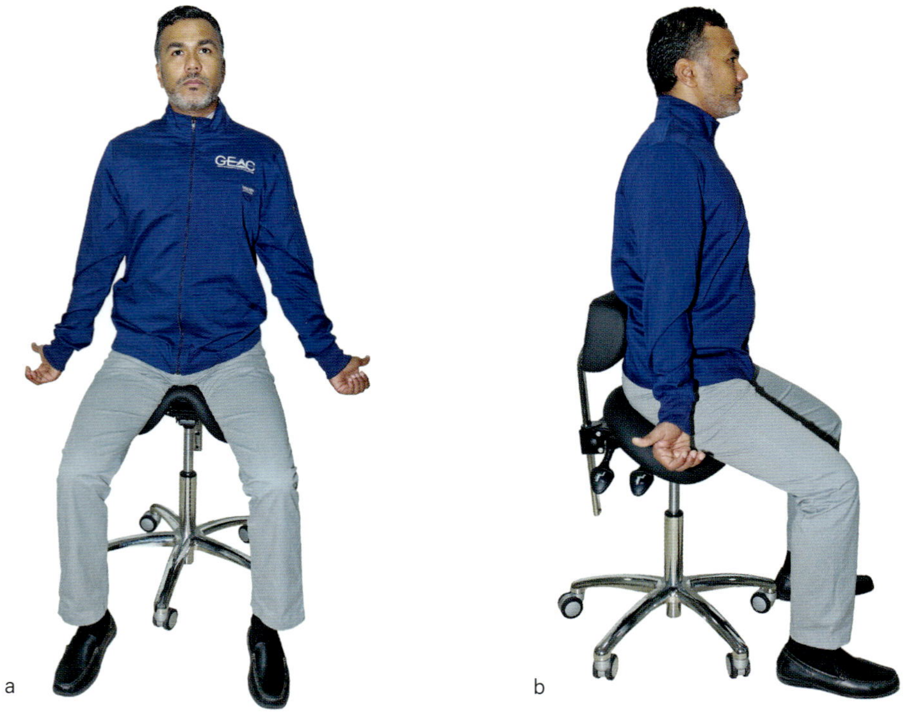

Chin tucks

A good way to create postural awareness to improve posture and decrease stress on your head, neck, and shoulders is a chin tuck exercise. Chin tucks are typically one of the key exercises recommended for keeping the head aligned above the spine, rather than drifting forward into poor posture. When done regularly and with proper form, chin tucks can help improve the strength, flexibility, and function of the neck.

Chin tucks can be performed while standing or sitting. A chin tuck is a movement of the head, pulling the chin with the head straight back until the stretch is felt. Hold for 5 seconds and repeat 10 times several times per day. This exercise will help the neck muscles reset the muscle memory in order to promote the neutral posture of cervical musculoskeletal tissues.[17]

Seated postural exercises

To create the best postural habits in the long term, the muscles involved in this posture must be trained. These mainly include the deep muscles of the back and abdominal muscles. This training should be combined with proper knowledge of the neutral position discussed earlier in this book. Ergonomist Bethany Valachi suggests the following exercise to improve postural awareness[18] (Fig 7-2):

- Sit in a seat that leans slightly downward or a saddle-type seat. Do not use the backrest at this time. Arch the back, and then flex or flatten it. Alternate between these two positions multiple times, and then find a position comfortable between the two.
- Maintain this position by pulling the navel inward toward your back. Keep this position throughout the exercise.
- Sit upright in the chair, raising your chest up.
- Stretch your head towards the ceiling, as if you had a spring attached to the back of your head pulling up.
- Take a deep breath and point your thumbs back (as in hitchhiking).
- Press the shoulder blades down together. Keep this position briefly.
- Allow your palms to turn inward and relax your sides while exhaling gently. Do not let the shoulders roll forward.
- Hold this position for at least 1 minute, then relax. Perform this exercise daily until this sitting posture becomes a habit.

Wall exercises

Another exercise to promote proper posture can be performed against the wall as follows[19]:

1. Position your feet 12 to 18 inches away from the wall with your knees slightly bent.
2. Lean back, placing your back against the wall.
3. Slowly press your lower back, tailbone, head, and shoulder blades against the wall. (If this causes pain or discomfort, relax until the pain goes away.)
4. Hold for 60 to 120 seconds, and perform this exercise several times per day.

Health and Fitness

Fitness is defined as the body's ability to function efficiently. In dental work, proper fitness can be very helpful to make the body resist long hours of awkward or sustained postures. Fitness can be divided into two areas: cardiorespiratory fitness and muscle fitness.

Cardiorespiratory fitness

Cardiorespiratory fitness is the first and most important type of fitness. The heart and the blood vessels transport oxygen from the lungs to the tissues. When oxygen is adequately transported, blood flow can more efficiently reach the organs and body systems. Blood is responsible for supplying nutrients and removing metabolic byproducts from the muscles. Among other effects, accumulation of these metabolic byproducts in the muscles makes them susceptible to syndromes such as tendonitis. On the other hand, adequate fitness of the cardiorespiratory system can help reduce stress and facilitate optimum performance.

Fitness experts and the American Heart Association recommend moderate physical exercises, performed at a maximum of 80% of the cardiac range, for approximately 30 minutes three or four times per week. Moderate workouts are preferable to vigorous workouts, because the latter aggressively engage muscle groups and generate fatigue in the body.[20]

Regular exercise increases health, reduces stress, and generates greater job satisfaction.

Regular exercise increases health, reduces stress, and generates greater job satisfaction. Another of its advantages is that it activates the movement of joints and bones, promoting contraction and muscular relaxation. These movements keep the joints lubricated for smooth and efficient ranges of motion and in turn allow the spinal discs to move and exchange fluids. The goal is to stretch and strengthen muscles and improve body condition.[21]

Muscle fitness

Muscle fitness plays a different role in body function. When operating at full capacity, there is a total resistance that muscles can handle. Improving the muscles allows the range of movement to be optimized. Poor positioning or injury reduces range and flexibility, "shrinking" the structures by shortening the tendons. This means range of motion becomes limited and you cannot reach as far.

With age comes muscle atrophy, diminishing strength and physical performance. It is believed that after the age of 35 years, we lose approximately 225 grams of muscle and gain about 600 grams of fat each year. All this contributes to a poor physical condition.[22]

Conclusion

Breaks and dynamic stretching can help prevent musculoskeletal disorders. Rest allows the body to heal from microtraumas caused by prolonged static posture, preventing fatigue, and exercise allows the muscles to get the nutrients they need and build strength. Your body is your greatest investment, and time should be devoted to giving it the care it needs. Short, frequent breaks are more effective than long, infrequent breaks. There are also specific stretches and exercises to help with postural awareness, which will allow you to maintain neutral posture throughout the day.

References

1. Rundcrantz BL, Johnsson B, Moritz U. Occupational cervico-brachial disorders among dentists. Analysis of ergonomics and locomotor functions. Swed Dent J 1991;15:105–115.
2. Marshall ED, Duncombe LM, Robinson RQ, Kilbreath SL. Musculoskeletal symptoms in New South Wales dentists. Aust Dent J 1997;42:240–246.
3. Bandy WD, Irion JM, Briggler M. The effect of static stretch and dynamic range of motion training on the flexibility of the hamstring muscles. J Orthop Sports Phys Ther 1998;27:295–300.
4. Westerblad H, Allen DG. Recent advances in the understanding of skeletal muscle fatigue. Curr Opin Rheumatol 2002;14:648–652.
5. University of North Carolina at Chapel Hill. Office Ergonomics. https://ehs.unc.edu/workplace-safety/ergonomics/office/. Accessed 31 March 2022.
6. Burton J; World Health Organization. WHO Healthy Workplace Framework and Model: Background and Supporting Literature and Practice. https://www.who.int/occupational_health/healthy_workplace_framework.pdf. Accessed 31 March 2022.
7. Karwowski W, Marras WS. The Occupational Ergonomics Handbook. Boca Raton, FL: CRC, 1999.
8. Shellock FG, Prentice WE. Warming-up and stretching for improved physical performance and prevention of sports-related injuries. Sports Med 1985;2:267–278.
9. Healthline. Stretching: 9 Benefits, Plus Safety Tips and How to Start. https://www.healthline.com/health/benefits-of-stretching. Accessed 31 March 2022.
10. Comes C, Valceanu AS, Rusu D, et al. A Study on the ergonomical working modalities using the dental operating microscope (DOM). Part II: Ergonomic design elements of the operating microscopes. Timisoara Medical J 2010;60:97–102.
11. Cailliet R. Soft Tissue Pain and Disability, ed 3. Philadelphia: F. A. Davis, 1996.
12. Harvard Health Publishing. Exercising to Relax. https://www.health.harvard.edu/staying-healthy/exercising-to-relax. Accessed 31 March 2022.
13. Cailliet R. Neck and Arm Pain, ed 3. Philadelphia: F. A. Davis, 1991.
14. The Back School. ERGO BREAK Wellness Sheets. https://thebackschool.net/ergo-break-wellness-sheets. Accessed 31 March 2022.
15. Van As GA. Digital documentation and the dental operating microscope: What you see is what you get. Int J Microdent 2009;1:30–41.
16. Page P. Current concepts in muscle stretching for exercise and rehabilitation. Int J Sports Phys Ther 2012;7:109–119.
17. Meyler Z. Easy Chin Tucks for Neck Pain. Spine-Health. https://www.spine-health.com/wellness/exercise/easy-chin-tucks-neck-pain. Accessed 31 March 2022.
18. Valachi B. Practice Dentistry Pain-Free: Evidence-Based Strategies to Prevent Pain and Extend Your Career. Portland, OR: Posturedontics, 2008.
19. Summit Orthopedics. Wall Posture. https://www.summitortho.com/services/back-neck-spine/treatments/spine-exercises-library/wall-posture/. Accessed 31 March 2022.
20. Mayo Clinic. Exercise Intensity: How to Measure It. https://www.mayoclinic.org/healthy-lifestyle/fitness/in-depth/exercise-intensity/art-20046887. Accessed 31 March 2022.
21. Pollack-Simon R. All the Right Moves: The Definitive Guide for Integrating Dental Team Ergonomics. Tulsa, OK: Pennwell, 2002.
22. Siparsky PN, Kirkendall DT, Garrett WE Jr. Muscle changes in aging: Understanding sarcopenia. Sports Health 2014;6:3640.

8

The Optical Microscope

The surgical microscope is the only tool in dentistry that allows the operator to improve vision and ergonomics in the same clinical act.

Chapter objectives

- **Understand how the microscope works and its benefits**
- **Learn how to adjust the microscope to achieve optimal posture**
- **Avoid the most frequent errors in using the microscope**
- **Learn about the available attachments that can be added to the microscope to improve ergonomics**

History of the Dental Microscope

Apotheker introduced the dental light microscope in 1981. The first microscope was poorly configured, and ergonomic use was difficult. It had only a single magnification (8×), foot support with insufficient balance, and straight eyepieces, and it was set at a focal length of 250 mm. This microscope also used angled instead of coaxial illumination, so it did not gain acceptance and was soon discontinued.[1]

In 1992, Gary Carr designed the first dental operating microscope, which would define the characteristics of the microscopes we use today:

- Coaxial lighting systems with high-intensity halogen or xenon lights
- Optics with magnification ranges adapted to the area of work (eg, 6×, 10×, 12×, 16×, and 20×)
- Tilting eyepieces
- Lighter systems, allowing optimal mobility to see any tooth or quadrant in the mouth[2]

The use of the surgical microscope in dentistry, especially in endodontics, has progressed from sporadic use in the early and mid 1990s to use by most endodontists today.[3] It became a necessity in endodontics due to the complexities of vision and small field of view, and it then spread to other dental disciplines such as restorative dentistry, prosthodontics, and periodontics.

The microscope is undoubtedly an essential tool for clinicians to learn—it has been a requirement in endodontic programs in the United States since

BOX 8-1 Glossary of terms

Field of view: Circular area that is observed when looking at the object under a certain magnification

Focal length: Distance between the optical center of the lens and focus (or focal point)

In focus: Phenomenon that occurs when reflected light spots from the object coincide with the focus of the lens

Out of focus: Phenomenon that occurs when light spots reflected by the object do not match the focus of the lens

Magnification: Quantity or degree of magnification of an object

Parfocalization: Balance between the camera and microscope (it is ideal to keep focus between both)

Focal plane: The plane on which the lens forms a sharp image, usually perpendicular to the optical axis

Depth of focus: Latitude of focus that materializes in the focal plane that can move from the true focal plane without reduction in the sharpness of the reproduced images

Image resolution: Ability to distinguish between two objects near each other and clearly differentiate them as separate and distinct

The microscope is undoubtedly an essential tool for clinicians to learn.

1998, and training may be required in other specialties as well. If all dentists can learn how to properly use the microscope, it will result in more predictable procedures while improving the health and professional longevity of the operator. Therefore, both the dentist and the patient benefit. It will be interesting to see what the future holds regarding training on this essential tool in dental schools.

Box 8-1 lists a glossary of terms associated with the optical microscope. To understand the magnification of the optical microscope, it is essential to understand the relationships between focal length, magnification, field of view, and depth of focus:

- The greater the focal length of the lens, the lower the final magnification.
- The lower the final magnification, the greater the field of view.
- The greater the field of view, the greater the depth of focus.
- The higher the magnification, the smaller the visual field.
- The higher the magnification, the shorter the depth of focus (image appears flatter).

Ergonomic Benefits of Microscopes

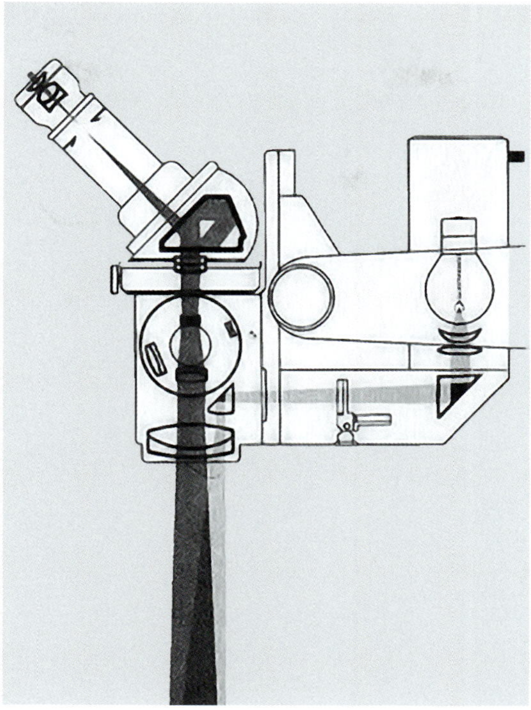

FIG 8-1 Coaxial lighting.

The microscope is a single solution to multiple problems in dentistry. It provides greater magnification for the dentist and also allows the operator to see by looking straight ahead in neutral posture, not inclining the head forward and straining the neck or back.[4]

In my personal opinion, the microscope should be promoted as an ergonomic tool as well as a magnification tool. An operator who has used the microscope for years and decides to perform a procedure with the naked eye or loupes will almost immediately begin feeling pain in the neck and back. Remember, your body is your greatest investment, and that should be enough reason to protect it with this great tool.

Integration of the microscope into any practice will require the addition of other synergistic ergonomic equipment for its use. This is because as the magnification increases, the depth and the diameter of the operative visual field decrease. In this sense, there is a greater demand to improve muscle and joint control (fingers and wrist), which may require stabilization of the thick motor joints (elbow and shoulder) with ergonomic stools[5] (see chapter 7).

Benefits of magnification

Users who have worked for years with loupes may feel no need to make a change to their processes. Loupes have many advantages—they are small, less expensive than microscopes, and have a minimal learning curve. Dentists who swear by loupes may feel that they can see at enough magnification and with adequate light.[6] However, if we compare conventional loupes with microscopes regarding working distance, there is approximately 35 cm from eyes to the patient's mouth with loupes and 54 cm with a microscope. This allows the head position with a microscope to be much more neutral. While there are now loupes on the market with a declination angle and focal distance that promote a more neutral head posture, microscopes allow five or more steps of magnification. Higher magnification can also help with the improvement of fine motor skills.[7] Loupes, on the other hand, have limited changes to magnification and consequently limited possibilities in what can be seen.[6] Another great difference is that coaxial lighting is used in the microscope, in which the light direction is the same as the optical direction (parallel to the visual axis), which is a crucial factor to get good depth of focus[8] (Fig 8-1). This stands in

TABLE 8-1 Visual information in optical microscope vs magnifying loupes[5]

Magnification	Visual information	Visual information compared with 2× loupes
Naked eye	1×	0.25×
2× loupes	4×	Even
3× loupes	9×	2.25×
4× loupes	16×	4×
6× microscope	36×	9×
10× microscope	100×	25×
20× microscope	400×	100×

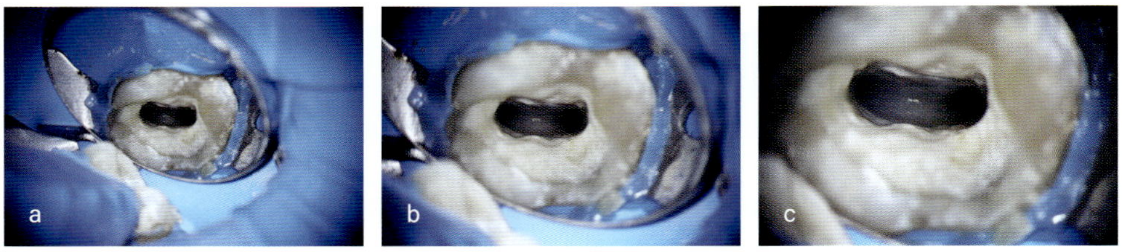

FIG 8-2 Microphotographs detailing the information obtained through different magnifications of the optical microscope: *(a)* 10×, *(b)* 16×, *(c)* 24×.

contrast to loupes, in which the light is not parallel to the axis of vision, which can generate shadows.[9] Personally, I consider loupes as the bridge of adaptation for the clinician's eyes to work with magnification before purchasing a microscope.

Magnification improves the outcome of clinical procedures because it allows for more precise surgery, resulting in less surgical trauma and better healing.[10] Dental procedures require professional skill and visual acuity, but they take place in a very small and dark work field. The microscope adds lighting and visual acuity, resulting in better quality of work. Studies on precision of treatment have shown that errors during procedures significantly decrease with built-in magnification.[4,11] The same studies showed that the inclusion of the microscope resulted in fewer mistakes than when magnifying loupes were used.[4,11]

Visual ability is enhanced with use of the operating light microscope, increasing the operator's ability to perform dental procedures with high precision.[12] Table 8-1 compares the visual information obtained with the microscope compared with loupes. This number is calculated by multiplying the number of horizontal pixels by the number of vertical pixels. For example, a 10× magnification microscope provides 25 times more information than that obtained through 2× magnifying loupes and more than 10 times that of 3× loupes[5] (Fig 8-2).

Carr[3] reported that without the aid of magnification, the human eye has the inherent ability to distinguish between two separate lines that are at least 200 μm (0.2 mm) apart. If lines are closer, the two objects will appear to be a single unit. Most people cannot focus at distances closer than 10 to 12 cm. To the extent that the eye-object distance (focal distance) decreases, the eyes must converge, which generates eye strain. This is the main disadvantage of dental practice without a microscope—the limitation of the eyes. Clinicians who work without magnification can perform 1- to 2-mm movements at a time.[13] At 20× magnification, refined movements can be as small as 10 to 20 μm at a time. The limitation in precision of movements and therefore treatment is not a limitation of the operator's hands but of their eyes.[13]

The limitation in precision of movements and therefore treatment is not a limitation of the operator's hands but of their eyes.

Also, as you get older, the ability to focus at closer distances is compromised, and the depth of field also decreases. Considering the uncomfortable situation of reduced proximity between the operator's face and the patient's, approaching closer is not a satisfactory solution. This is the biggest ergonomic problem that dentists face. Having said this, the microscope solves both concerns in a single clinical act due to its ability to magnify the image in several steps, in shadow-free coaxial light, and with the objective lens producing a fixed focal length (200–300 cm) or a variable focal length that allows continuous zoom from 200 to 400 cm, allowing the operator to position themselves in a position close to neutral. Alternatively, an optical microscope can increase the resolution limit mentioned previously from 0.2 mm to 0.006 mm. Therefore, with magnification, the resolution of the human eye improves enormously. In addition, having five to six levels of magnification available, from 2× to 26×, lighting becomes an essential component to increase the visualization.

It is no secret that dentistry is a profession with a high demand for visual requirements and precision in both diagnosis and treatment, and it is also no longer a secret how the use of the microscope helps to improve the motor skills to perform high-quality procedures.[7,14]

Benefits to posture

The introduction of the microscope to the dental office has been a great innovation that has generated many ergonomic changes. Most of the microscope work is done under indirect vision, which allows an improvement in the operator's posture.[15] Current optical microscopes are integrated with a source of coaxial light that allows an unobstructed illumination free from shadows in the operative field. This provides better visualization in the oral cavity, even in those areas that are most difficult to access. The light intensity and color temperature approximate those of natural sunlight, which improves the definition of the visual field.

Biomechanically, the operator must reach forward from the trunk or head to be able to see. The focal distance is limited in the naked eye, and the microscope solves this problem. Without a microscope, there is no possibility to see unless you reach about 30 cm from the patient's mouth. But with the microscope, we can remain at a distance of about 50 cm from the mouth.

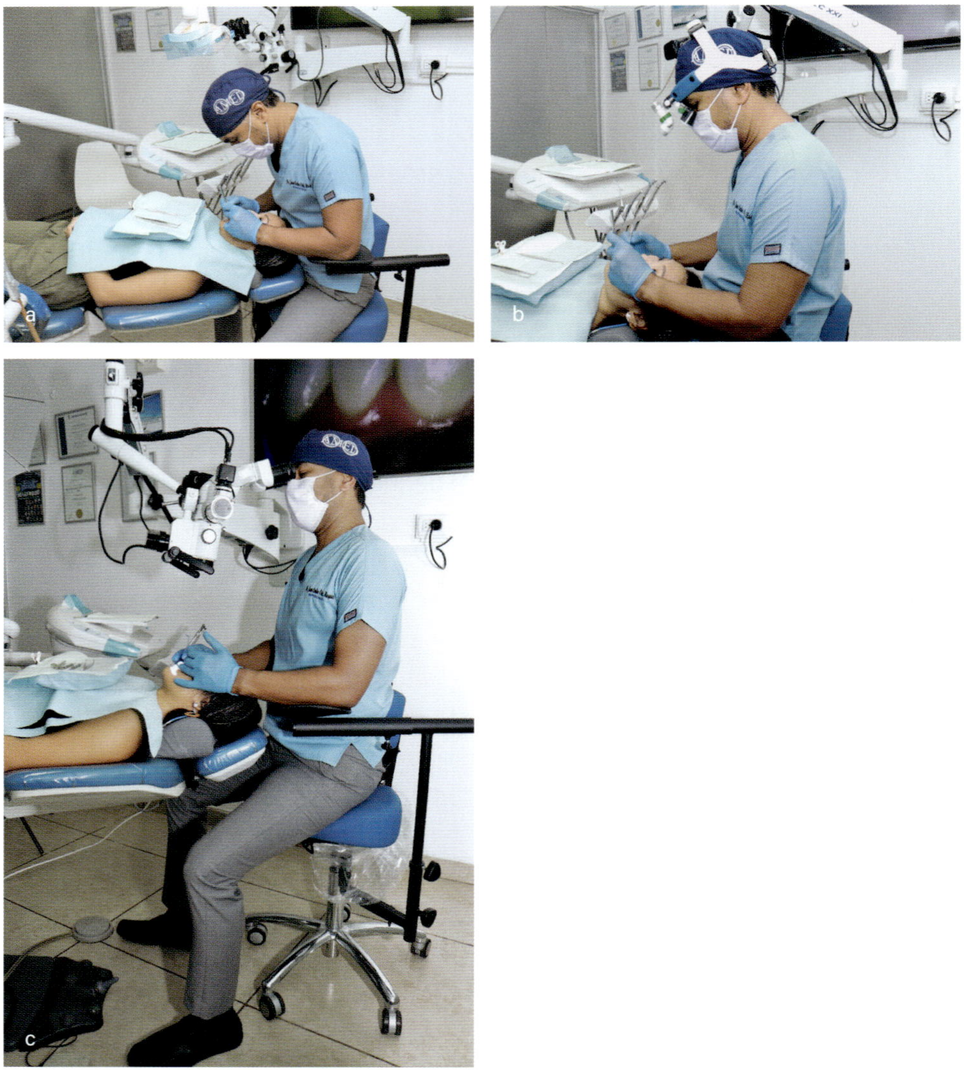

FIG 8-3 *(a)* Poor posture with naked-eye dentistry; the back and head are tilted forward. *(b)* Slightly improved but still poor posture with loupes; the back is straight but the neck is still bent. *(c)* Correct, upright posture with the microscope.

The operating microscope allows the dentist to sit in an upright position, closer to the neutral and balanced posture (Fig 8-3). Using the microscope promotes working in a posture with the head up rather than bent up to 20 degrees. The line of vision remains horizontal. This balanced neutral position obtained through the microscope has been very useful to prevent ergonomic problems that may cause job-related musculoskeletal disorders in dentists.[2] In addition to maintaining an upright posture, it prevents fatigue, tension, and stress on the neck and lower back, allowing the dentist to focus completely on their hands. The microscope enables the retina to focus 100% on the desired area, avoiding eye fatigue. This is also helped by the previously mentioned coaxial lighting, which prevents shadows from forming and making it more difficult to see.[16]

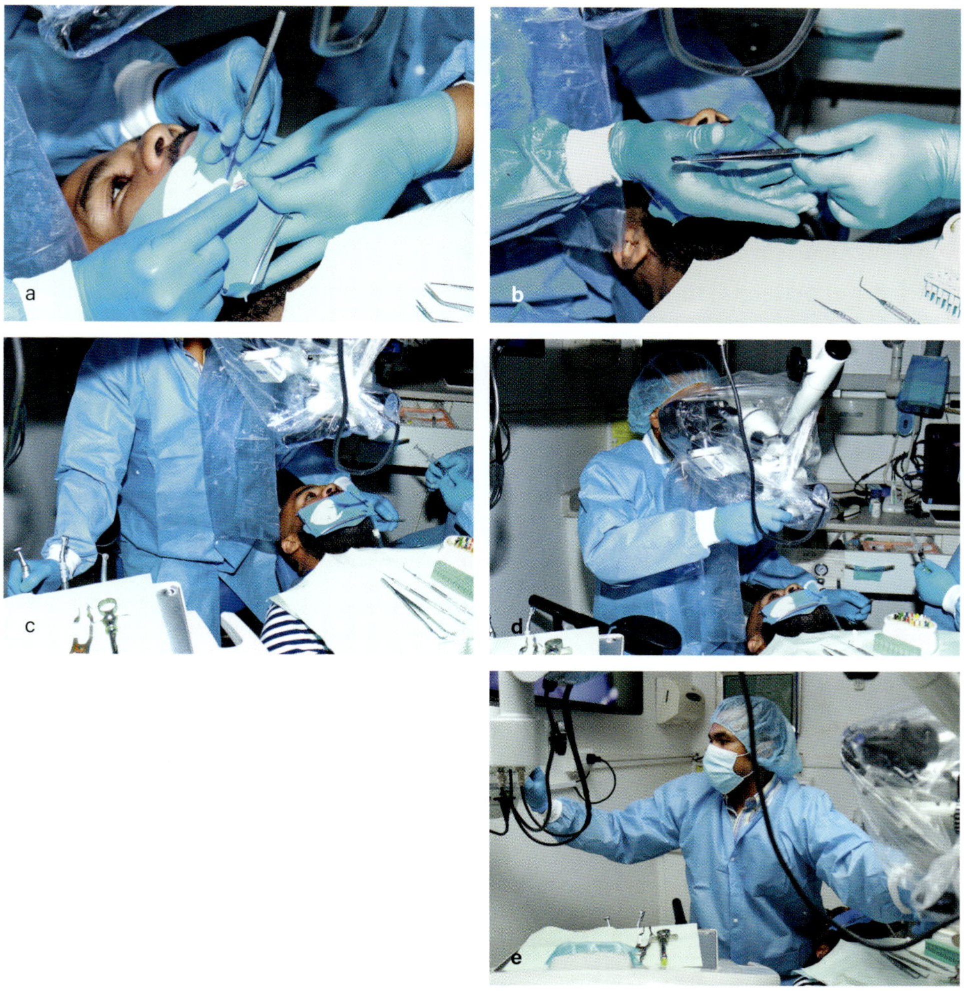

FIG 8-4 Laws of movement: finger, hand, and wrist movements in different procedures. *(a)* Class I movement: fingers. *(b)* Class II movement: wrist and fingers. *(c)* Class III movement: elbow, wrist, and fingers. *(d)* Class IV movement: movement originated from the shoulder. *(e)* Class V movement: movement that includes rotation from the waist.[9]

Classes of movement

To understand the efficient workflow using a microscope, you must understand the basic principles of ergonomic movements, divided into five classes[9] (Fig 8-4):

1. Class I: Movement of the fingers only
2. Class II: Movement of the fingers and wrist only
3. Class III: Movement that originates from the elbow
4. Class IV: Movement that originates from the shoulder
5. Class V: Movement that includes rotation and inclination from the waist

All equipment should be within arm's reach.

During a dental procedure, movement for both the dentist and the assistant should remain within Classes I to III—preferably Classes I and II. All equipment should be within arm's reach. The assistant should be properly trained to hand instruments to the operator so they can stay focused on the field of view while working with a microscope. The assistant can follow along with the procedure through a monitor, seeing when to provide suction and transfer instruments.

Learning how to use the microscope

In addition to being a mostly ergonomic tool, the microscope is a magnification tool. One of the greatest obstacles when learning to use this tool is to adapt the eyes and hands to the different magnification steps. The different magnifications result in loss or gain in the visual field, depth of focus, lighting, and image resolution. An understanding of these components is essential to choose the proper magnification for a given procedure. Sometimes we need to see in depth, and sometimes we need to see structural references in neighboring teeth and tissues. Knowing how to adjust what you will see will ensure a seamless and efficient workflow at all times.

One of the main limitations in the incorporation of this technology in dentistry is the learning curve to adapt your hands and eyes to work better and faster. Proper training is necessary to develop habits, and habits develop a healthy practice.[17] Currently, there are many training centers in the world available to professionals who wish to train and improve with this excellent tool. Mastering the use of the microscope requires time; thus, the trainings are sometimes long. However, this is necessary so that the professional can really master the microscope and overcome the learning curve. Taking a hands-on course will put the dentist on the right track to use this technology properly, but only daily use will guarantee the flow and comfort we need in clinical practice to get to the point of frequent use during treatments, which of course is the main goal.

Choosing a Microscope

There are several important factors when purchasing a microscope, which affect both ergonomics and performance of the microscope:

- Image quality
- Depth of focus in the image
- Mechanical strength
- Maneuverability and smooth movements
- Compatibility with other brands
- Magnification factors
- Versatility in models and stands
- Support and technical service
- Warranty

Because the microscope is a large instrument that will take up space, it becomes necessary to plan the organization of the office around it. Using the services of a professional architect or designer—or even consulting a colleague who uses a microscope in their practice—can help you make the best decision. This will ensure that the operatory is of the best dimensions to accommodate the microscope and that the best design of microscope for your office (ie, floor stand, wall-mounted, or ceiling-mounted) can be selected.

For example, if you are starting a practice from scratch or performing a remodel and wish to use a wall-mounted microscope, this will dictate where to build the walls of the room and where to mount the cabinets. Everything should be strategically planned for maximum ease and comfort for the operator and other staff. While using the microscope, the operator must not take their eyes off the eyepieces or take their hands out of the operating field to reach the instruments; the operator must always keep contact with the patient's mouth, and instruments must always be in contact with your fingers, following the concept of minimum horizontal reach.

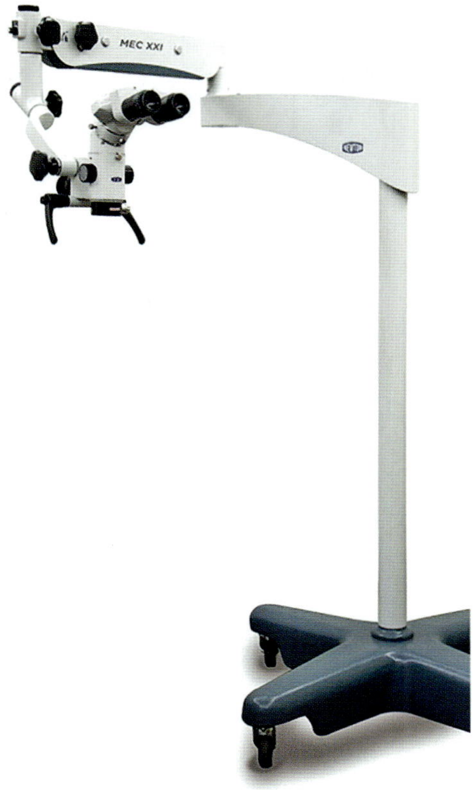

FIG 8-5 Optical microscope with foot stand.

In recent years, 3D microscopes have become available. The difference with these microscopes is that there are no eyepieces. This ensures that the surgeon practices in an upright working posture while keeping visual contact with the surgical field and the surrounding area. It allows for comfort, freedom of movement, less eye fatigue, and unobstructed peripheral vision.

Types of stands and mounts

It is essential that the microscope is stable while working. The ease of maneuverability is an important ergonomic factor to consider when acquiring the microscope. It should stay balanced when adding accessories like a beam splitter, photo and video elbow, reflex cameras, video camera, and eyepiece extender, among others. These add-ons will add weight to the microscope arm, and if it is not sturdy enough, the extra weight will set the microscope off balance, losing focal length and focus—possibly in the midst of a procedure. At worst, this can result in a mistake or harm to the patient; at best, it will cause a disruption to the workflow. The type of stand chosen will therefore depend on the available space within the operatory.

Foot stand

This type of stand (Fig 8-5) is ideal when the ceiling is very high, the dental chair is not close to any walls, or the walls or ceiling are not built to support the weight of the microscope (35 kg for the wall or 44 kg for the ceiling). Its main advantages are that it can be moved to multiple offices and does not need to be fixed to any surface. A disadvantage is that the large base (usually between 2 and 2.5 square feet) takes up floor space that may be limited. If the office is small and there is

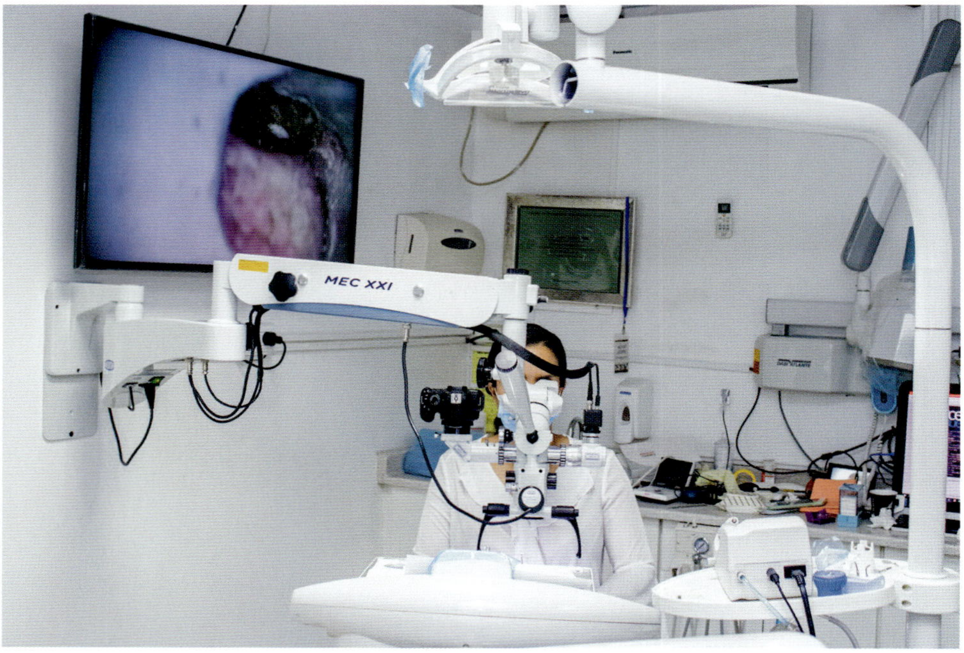

FIG 8-6 Optical microscope with wall mount.

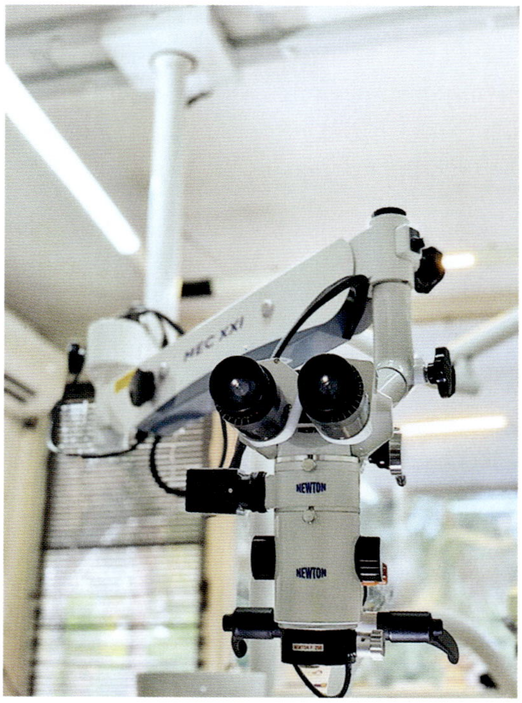

FIG 8-7 Microscope mounted from the ceiling.

not much room for staff to move around the microscope and reach other instruments, this will cause ergonomic problems rather than solving them.

Wall mount

This is a very functional setup for most clinics (Fig 8-6). Because it is attached to the wall, the microscope can be put out of the way while not in use, allowing staff to move around freely. Of course, when it is in use, it will block off space between the wall and the patient—usually on the operator's right-hand side. In addition, the walls of the operatory must have been engineered to withstand the weight of the mount.

From an ergonomic standpoint, the ceiling mount is the best recommendation.

Ceiling mount

The ceiling mount is ideal because it allows for the most freedom of movement around the operatory regardless of whether the microscope is in use (Fig 8-7). From an ergonomic standpoint, this is the best recommendation. However, the ceiling must be able to support the weight.

Light sources

As mentioned, the coaxial light parallel with the operator's axis of vision is one of the great advantages of the microscope for generating illuminated working fields. Good lighting is indispensable in dentistry because the work is carried out in dark and narrow cavities. Quantity and quality of light in the working field are as important as magnification.[18] Increasing the light levels can increase the apparent resolution. The appropriate light provides the operator with a greater diagnostic capacity and the ability to carry out the work in greater detail, without having to lean forward from the trunk or neck to see.

Microscopes may have the following different types of light:

- *Halogen:* Provides a 2300 Kelvin artificial yellow light. It is not recommended for quality documentation.
- *Xenon:* Provides daylight-type white light at 5000 Kelvin with 500 hours of life.
- *LED:* Provides white light at 5300 to 6500 Kelvin, very similar to xenon light but with the advantage of 50,000 to 70,000 hours of useful life.[19]

When recording, the amount of light is key to obtaining clear images with appropriate exposure and depth of field. Documentation with photo or video is one of the great benefits of microscope dentistry, which allows the best communication between patient and dentist, with other colleagues, and for legal records.[10]

Accessories

Accessories are available as attachments to the microscope to enhance ergonomics by providing greater economy of movement, maneuverability in hard-to-reach areas, controls that are easier to reach, and more. All the mentioned accessories that we can add to the microscope facilitate easy use and smooth movements. They make it possible to maneuver the equipment while working and promote ergonomic positioning of the operator and assistant as well as an efficient workflow.

Eyepiece extender

This is an optical element that is placed between the eyepieces and the body of the microscope that aims to bring the eyepieces closer to the operator's eyes (Fig 8-8). It is essential for ergonomics because it prevents forward head movement. It is made in angulations ranging from 30 to 45 degrees, depending on the brand of microscope.

VarioFocus lens

This is an objective lens that provides an expanded field of view and magnification range while keeping the microscope in the same position. Most of these lenses come with 200 to 400 mm of multifocal distance, which is a versatile way to allow the working distances to be extended. This accessory allows a tall or short operator to use the same microscope without altering their neutral working posture by having a wide working distance. It is undoubtedly one of the most ergonomic accessories that currently exists in the dental microscope market and also helps to flatten the learning curve when adapting to a microscope because of its ease of use.

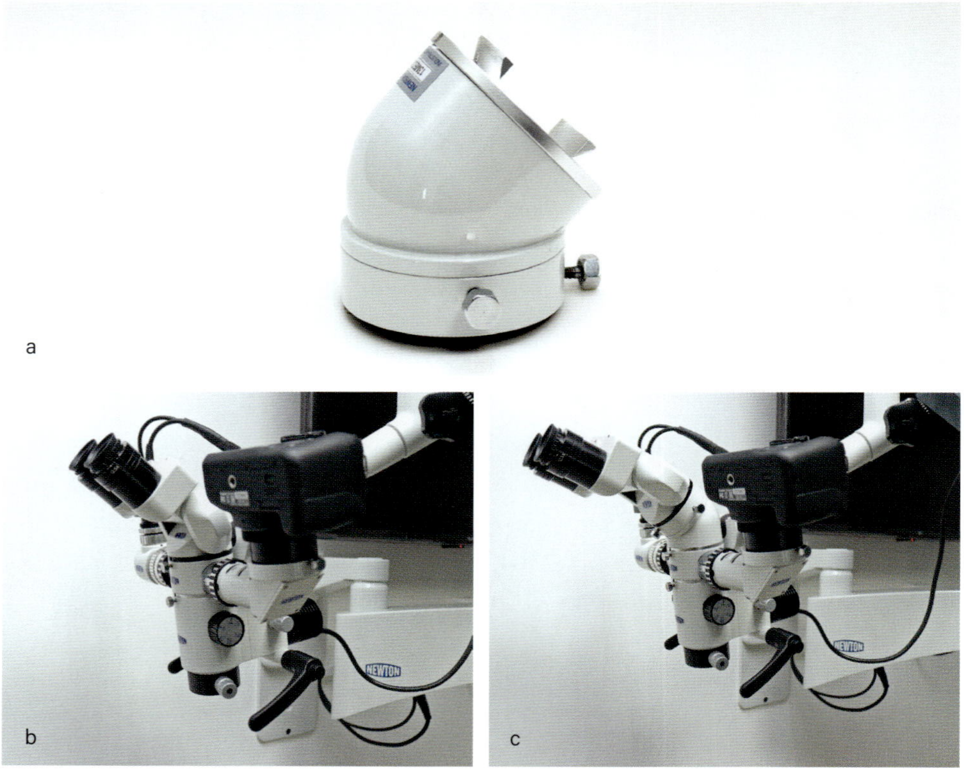

FIG 8-8 *(a)* Eyepiece extender. *(b)* Microscope without extender installed. *(c)* Microscope with extender installed.

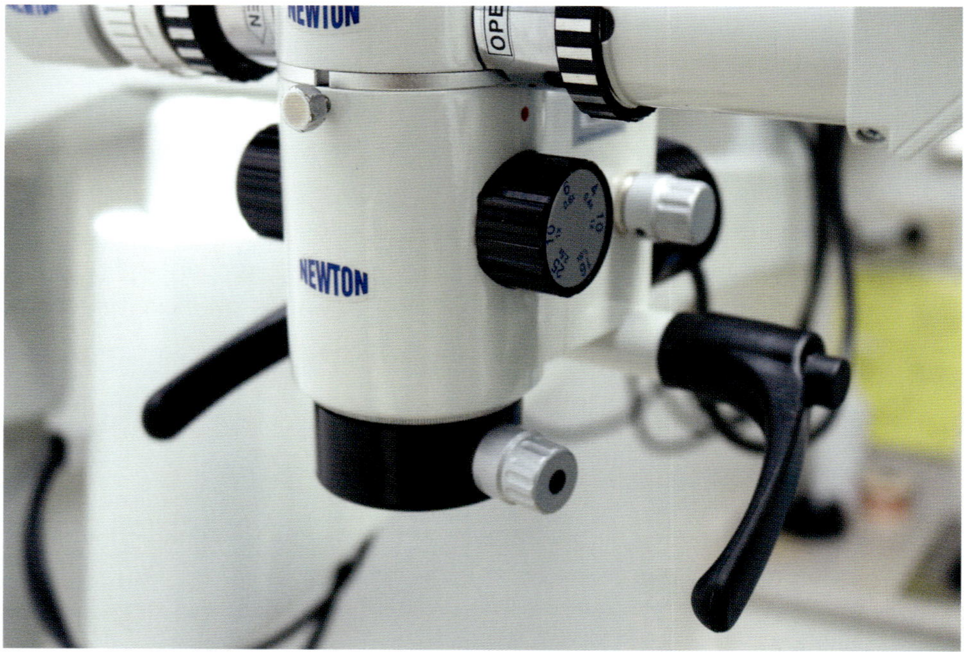

FIG 8-9 Micro focus system of the microscope.

Micro focus system

The micro focus system is an accessory placed within the objective lens of the microscope (Fig 8-9). It is fundamental for ergonomics because it allows an in-depth focus up to 20 mm, which makes it possible to keep the microscope in position and gain depth focus without raising or lowering the whole body of the microscope.

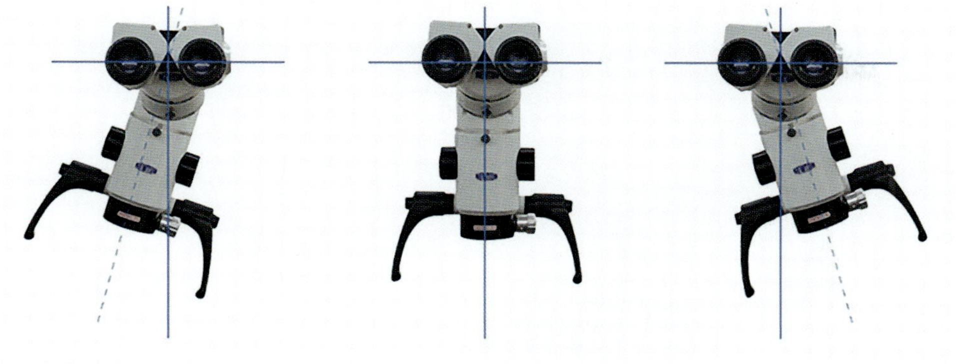

FIG 8-10 Interface for pendulum movements.

Interface for pendulum movements of the microscope body (rotary ring)

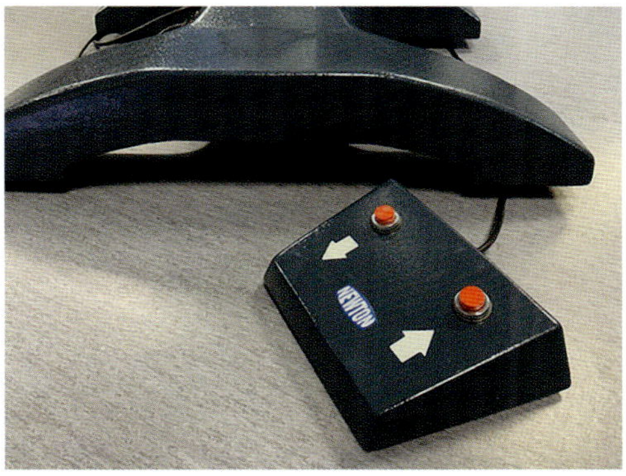

FIG 8-11 Foot control.

This type of interface, which is placed between the eyepiece and the body of the microscope, allows simple and precise movements. It provides a constant straight viewing position through the eyepieces, regardless of the angle of the body of the microscope, and enables the operator to maintain straight posture without taking their eyes off the object (Fig 8-10). It also prevents neck and trunk rotations. It is highly functional in fields such as restorative dentistry, periodontics, surgery, and prosthodontics, in which the operator must constantly move to various surfaces of the tooth.

Handgrip for balance and brake

Handgrips use magnetic clutches, allowing the operator to easily maneuver to the desired working position. A handgrip also allows additional accessories such as a co-observation tube and photo adapter to be simultaneously connected.

Foot controls

The pedal control allows the microscope to be moved using the feet rather than the hands. This enables the operator to focus exclusively on the movement of their fingers and hands in the operative act performed (Fig 8-11).

Handle controls

Light and zoom control from the handles, which are located in positions close to the operator's hands, are ergonomically relevant because they allow for relatively short

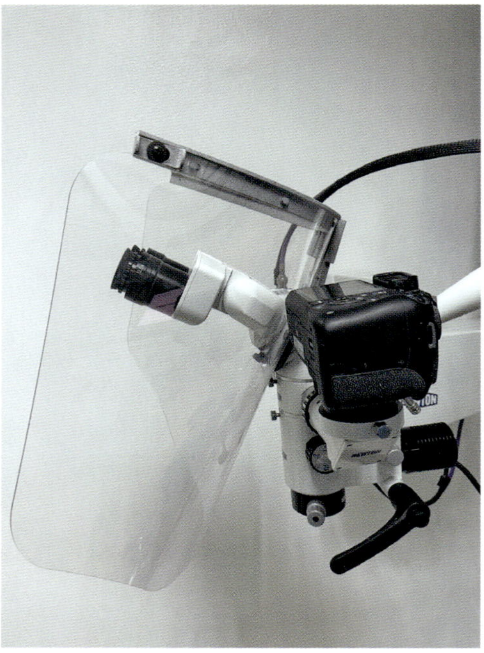

FIG 8-12 Shield to protect the operator.

movements. This prevents fatigue of some muscles and in turn improves workflow. The most expensive and sophisticated microscopes on the market will provide these options.

Safety barriers

Ergonomics is also about safety. Although the microscope moves us an additional 20 cm away from the patient's mouth compared to the naked eye, it also requires an adequate protection or barrier to avoid cross-contamination. Infection control is not only about patient-to-patient contamination. Shields and barriers have been developed especially for the microscope (Fig 8-12). These can be used on a daily basis in clinical practice.

Proper Positioning in Microscope Dentistry

To maintain proper posture and microscope orientation, positioning must occur systematically, as follows:

1. Operator position
2. Patient position
3. Microscope position

Position is everything in dentistry, and by respecting this sequence, the dentist and assistant will always be able to achieve an efficient and comfortable workflow. Changes to this sequence promote nonneutral postures and increase interruptions while managing the microscope and instruments around the working field in four-handed dentistry.[21]

Operator position

The operator is the center point of the entire system and office. All the components—patient chair, stools, counter, materials, and instruments—should conform to the operator's comfort to produce the best clinical result and keep them healthy and productive in the long term. Consider your comfort throughout the procedure, maintaining postural awareness at all times. The assistant can provide support in this area as well by pointing out any postural deviations.

First, the operator's back must be kept straight, and the light of the microscope must remain perpendicular to the floor. To reduce the amount of stress of the operator, the best position ranges between 11 and 12 o'clock. The 12 o'clock position is the most ergonomic position to treat the four quadrants of the mouth with indirect vision. It also allows you to be closer to the assistant and properly seated in an ergonomic stool while using the microscope and achieving the maximum musculoskeletal support.[21–23]

The operator is the center point of the entire system and office.

Patient position

Once the operator is correctly positioned, the patient can be positioned. The position of the patient is an undervalued consideration, but it shouldn't be. Mispositioning of the patient causes a domino effect that will result in mispositioning of the microscope and discomfort for the entire work system. It is a common mistake to ensure the patient's comfort above all else. Of course, we do want our patients to be comfortable for the procedure, but not at the expense of the operator or the assistant. The patient is in this position for a short while; the staff are in these positions all day, every day.

Conscious and systematic positioning of the patient facilitates ergonomic work in all quadrants of the patient's mouth on any of the tooth surfaces. Together with the use of the mirror for indirect vision, it will allow the operator versatility when working actively inside the patient's mouth, whether for prosthetic preparations, endodontics, or surgery.

Positioning the patient horizontally in the dental chair will greatly facilitate the patient's mouth being in the most strategic visual position, just under the light of the microscope.[24] The patient's head should be placed at the end of the headrest, with a minimal amount of space between their head and the operator's body (see chapter 6). The operator should direct the patient to the correct position with verbal instruction.

The patient can also be directed in the following ways if the operator needs to focus on a particular area of the mouth:

- To work on molars, the patient is asked to raise the chin upward.
- To work on mandibular incisors and premolars, the patient is asked to bring the chin toward the chest.
- To work in proximal, vestibular, or palatal/lingual areas, the patient is asked to turn the head laterally. The operator can use their hands to guide the patient's head if necessary.

Remember, it is always preferable for the patient to turn their head to give you the best access than for you to turn your head in a nonneutral way.

It is possible to have a situation where the patient cannot tolerate certain positions. Patients with chronic muscular disorders, those with a tendency to dizziness, or elderly patients may not be able to recline fully. In this situation, work with the patient to get them to a position as close to horizontal as possible so they can withstand the procedure while allowing the best possible posture for the operator.[25] It may also be helpful to provide the patient with a cervical or lumbar pillow for additional support.

The chair height should be adjusted so the patient's mouth is at the same height or slightly higher than the operator's elbows (relaxed on either side of the body) to promote neutral elbow, forearm, wrist, and hand working postures.[26]

Key aspects of patient positioning therefore include the following:

- The patient should be placed horizontally on the dental chair.
- The patient's head should be at the end of the headrest.
- Use verbal indications depending on the tooth and quadrant being worked on.
- The height of the patient's mouth should be at the level of the operator's elbows when relaxed on either side of the body or slightly higher.
- Positioning should be systematic.

Microscope position

After controlling our position in the ergonomic stool and the patient's in the dental chair, it is time to place the microscope in working position for the task at hand. The diopters in the eyepieces must be adjusted individually according to the dominant eye as well as the interpupillary distance to achieve the correct focus of the microscope and to be able to observe clearly through the eyepieces at all times. The operator should not tilt the head forward more than 20 degrees at any point during the procedure[26] (see Fig 8-3c). The eyepieces may be tilted 100 to 120 degrees in relation to the body of the microscope. If they are tilted at only 90 degrees or more than 120 degrees, this may promote nonneutral flexion or hyperextension of the neck.

The body of the microscope should be directly perpendicular to the floor or slightly forward, inclined 0 to 15 degrees. This will maintain the proper inclination of the eyepieces with respect to the operator's neutral head posture. A good reference when working with the microscope is for the operator to get as close as possible to the patient's head, then to bring the microscope to the operator's position. The operator should not need to lean toward the microscope. Bringing the microscope to the operator, and not the other way around, will prioritize neutral posture from the start. Because of how modern microscopes are designed, the working distance can easily be ergonomically managed when the patient's mouth is at the height of the operator's elbows or slightly higher. The microscope will allow the appropriate magnification level to be easily selected. Box 8-2 lists ergonomic recommendations for how to adjust the microscope.

It is essential that the area of work be in proper focus. By making a parfocal adjustment, once the object is in focus, the focus will remain even when the magnification is changed.[27] This is usually done at the highest magnification and should be performed at the start of treatment. Otherwise, there will be multiple interruptions to the procedure to move the microscope and refocus every time the magnification is changed. This causes both physical and mental fatigue with repetitive movements.

Bringing the microscope to the operator, and not the other way around, will prioritize neutral posture from the start.

BOX 8-2 Ergonomic recommendations for adjusting the microscope

- The eyepieces of the microscope should range from 100 to 120 degrees in angulation.
- The body of the microscope should be straight, perpendicular to the floor, or inclined slightly forward from 0 to 15 degrees.
- With the head in neutral posture, the microscope should be brought to the operator's eyes.
- The patient's mouth should be at the same height as the operator's elbows or up to 2 cm higher to approximate the focal distance.

TABLE 8-2 Most frequent errors when using the microscope in dentistry

Ergonomic problem	Error in microscope use
Neck flexion	• The eyepieces are tilted at more than 120 degrees. • The dental chair, patient, and body of the microscope are placed too low.
Neck hyperextension	• The eyepieces are tilted at 90 degrees. • The dental chair, patient, and body of the microscope are placed too high.
Trunk-neck rotation	• The working position is in the wrong clock direction. • The dental chair has a large backrest with fins that does not allow the dentist to get close enough to the patient's mouth. • The patient's head is in an inappropriate position. • The delivery system is too far behind the operator. • The operator is working without an assistant.
Arm abduction	• The operator is using a nonergonomic stool or one without an armrest. • The operator is working without an assistant. • Instruments and handpieces are too far away for horizontal reach.

Mistakes in positioning

Although the microscope is a great tool that can facilitate neutral working posture for the operator, mistakes can be made with its use that will interfere with these benefits (Table 8-2). A proper understanding of biomechanics and good posture habits can help you avoid these mistakes.

The surgical microscope is an innovative technology that helps align the operator's neck and back, bringing them closer to neutral working posture—but it cannot guarantee this posture if it is not complemented by education and training of the operator. The errors mentioned here are the result of a deficiency in information and training, but they can easily be resolved by efficient, sequential positioning. By completing these steps, the dentist and the assistant can achieve a healthy, comfortable, stress-free working environment. Procedures will be done with greater precision and more certainty because the dentist will receive much more visual information than can be attained with the naked eye.

Improper magnification

It can be tempting to use the highest magnification possible to focus on a single point, but this will limit the amount of information that the dentist can perceive. Remember: The higher the magnification, the smaller the visual field. A too-small visual field can lead you to miss anatomical reference points, surrounding tissues, the axial axis of the tooth to be treated, and more. At higher magnifications, the focus will be concentrated in a single point, while the periphery may be blurred. The loss of this peripheral information can be frustrating because it can be very important.

Remember: The higher the magnification, the smaller the visual field.

Our best recommendation is to work at low magnifications when actively working, whether with high- or low-speed handpieces, suturing, using the scalpel in surgical procedures, carving for restorations, and in restorative procedures. Medium and maximum magnification can be used for details and inspection. With practice over time, our hands become more skilled, and we are able to actively execute more procedures in intermediate magnifications where there is greater visual magnification and perimeter references.

Improper use of the mirror

The other factor that limits the fluid use of the microscope is not using the mirror in indirect vision. Correct use of the mirror will allow always working in a neutral position with the microscope in the areas or on surfaces that are more difficult to access safely and comfortably.[28]

The further away work is done from the medial plane of your body, the greater the fatigue. Working near the center of mass of the body puts the body on the optimal path to health.[29] The area of focus should be completely centered in the mirror during the procedure. This can be accomplished with micromovements such as moving the mirror and macromovements such as moving the patient's head.

Neck flexion

Flexion is the movement by which the bones or other parts of the body approach each other in anteroposterior direction, parallel to the sagittal plane. It is a consequence of the contraction of one or more muscle flexors. In dentistry under a microscope, neck flexion occurs as a result of factors having to do with working distance errors: specifically, by placing the body of the microscope very low, placing the eyepieces at an angle greater than 120 degrees, or positioning the dental chair very low (see Table 8-2). This directly affects the posture of the operator in order to "see" the working field. When positioning the patient or microscope very low, the dentist's neck must be placed into flexion, often creating a line of sight at more than 20 degrees below the horizon line. For a long procedure, maintaining postures like this below the horizon line could be harmful to the neck muscles and promote painful syndromes in the area (Fig 8-13).

Neck hyperextension

Anatomically, *extension* is a movement of separation between bones or parts of the body in the anteroposterior direction. It is opposite to flexion. Placing the microscope and dental chair very high and placing the eyepieces at 90 degrees could cause this

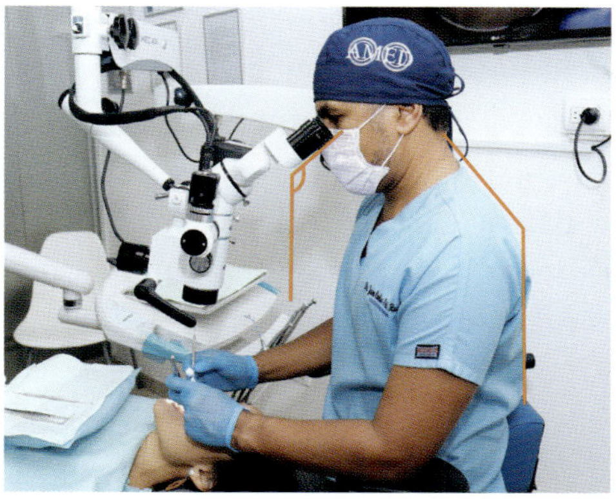

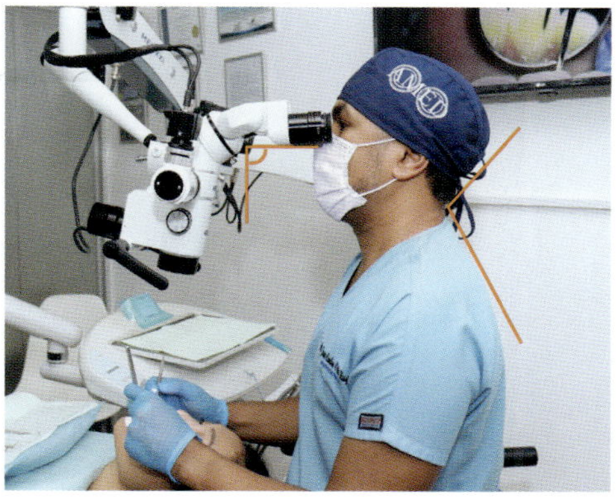

FIG 8-13 *(left)* Because the patient is positioned too low, the microscope is at a great angle, causing neck flexion in the operator.

FIG 8-14 *(right)* Here the microscope is positioned too high, causing too short of an angle of the eyepieces and resulting in neck hyperextension in the operator.

kind of bad posture (Fig 8-14), in which the head is extended, creating tension in the neck and shoulder muscles. If this is done frequently or for prolonged periods of time, it can be responsible for painful syndromes in the area.

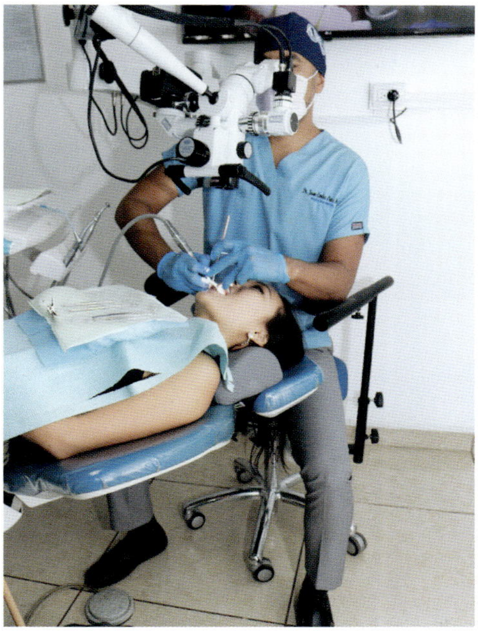

FIG 8-15 Even with a microscope, the operator is abducting his arm, elevating his shoulder, and experiencing trunk torsion and neck rotation.

Arm abduction

Abduction is the movement by which a part of the body moves away from to the medial plane of symmetry (transverse plane). Arm abduction is very common in dentistry, with or without a microscope. Not working with an assistant promotes movement from the shoulder to reach instruments or work equipment. Likewise, the placement of frequent-use supplies, instruments, and equipment away from the work area forces horizontal reaching motions toward the area. Armrests allow movement without abduction by supporting the weight of the arms. Abduction can generate musculoskeletal disorders such as cuff rotator impingement and, to a lesser extent, trapezius myalgia (see chapter 4).

Torsion/rotation of neck and trunk

Rotation is the movement or change of orientation; in this case, it refers to a part of the body in reference to the axis of rotation. In dentistry, it occurs both with and without magnification due to positioning errors. For example, if the operator is located on the side opposite the working field and does not guide the patient to move their head laterally, the operator's neck and torso will rotate to gain access to the working area.

Torsion and rotation of the neck and trunk also occur when instruments are positioned behind the operator when working without an assistant. If these movements are performed frequently and for prolonged periods of time, it will increase the tendency to develop musculoskeletal syndromes (Fig 8-15).

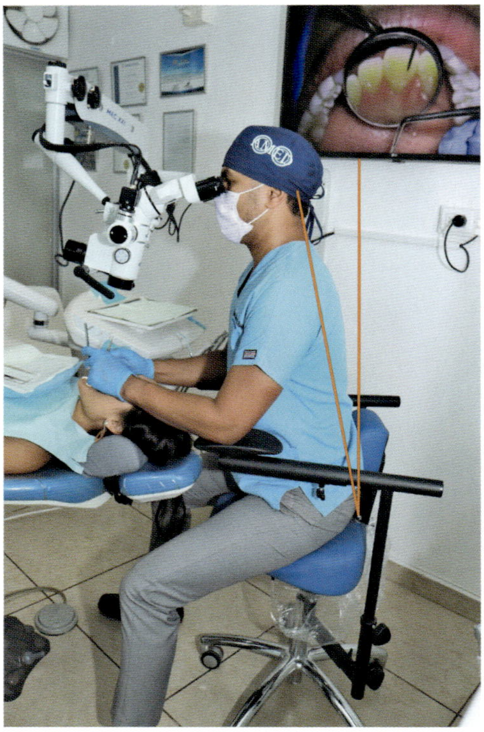

FIG 8-16 Forward trunk posture.

Forward trunk flexion

Although this occurs to a lesser extent, its impact on the spinal discs is relevant. It usually occurs due to the patient's improper positioning in the dental chair. When the patient does not place their head at the end of the headrest, it generates extra distance between the mouth and the microscope. This can only be solved by moving the microscope forward and as a result leaning the head and the trunk forward from the lumbar spine (Fig 8-16). This can be easily corrected by asking the patient to move to the edge of the headrest. In turn, the microscope has an attachment called the eyepiece extender that allows the eyepieces to move closer to the operator rather than the other way around, which allows a better posture of the head and neck (see Fig 8-8).

Conclusion

Using an optical microscope is one of the foundations of ergonomic dentistry. It allows the operator to maintain the best and most neutral head posture in a way that cannot be achieved with naked-eye dentistry or loupes. The microscope has the added benefit of allowing procedures to be performed with greater precision, helping the patient as well as the dentist. There is a learning curve to incorporating the microscope into clinical practice, but many training programs and courses are available. When purchasing a microscope, consideration should be given to the type of stand or mount that will be used, the type of lighting available for the microscope, as well as the accessories to enhance the microscope. The operator, patient, and microscope should be systematically positioned to allow the operator to reap all the benefits of the microscope.

References

1. Apotheker H, Jako GJ. A microscope for use in dentistry. J Microsurg 1981;3:7–10.
2. Kim S, Kratchman S. Modern endodontic surgery concepts and practice: A review. J Endod 2006;32:601–623.
3. Carr GB. Microscopes in endodontics. J Calif Dent Assoc 1992;20(11):55–61.
4. Zaugg B, Stassinakis A, Hotz P. Influence of magnification tools on the recognition of simulated preparation and filling errors [in German]. Schweiz Monatsschr Zahnmed 2004;114:890–896.

5. Van As GA. Extreme Magnification and Laser Dentistry: Seeing the Light. Dental Academy of Continuing Education.
6. Kamath D, Paul J, Joseph A, Varghese J. Magnification in endodontics: Dental loupes vs microscope. J Odont Rest 2015;3:31–34.
7. Bowers DJ, Glickman GN, Solomon ES, He J. Magnification's effect on endodontic fine motor skills. J Endod 2010;36:1135–1138.
8. Perrin P, Neuhaus KW, Eichenberger M, Lussi A. Influence of different loupe systems and their light source on the vision in endodontics. Swiss Dent J 2019;129:922–928.
9. Carr GB, Murgel CA. The use of the operating microscope in endodontics. Dent Clin North Am 2010;54:191–214.
10. Michaelides PL. Use of the operating microscope in dentistry [published correction appears in J Calif Dent Assoc 1996;24(10):9]. J Calif Dent Assoc 1996;24(6):45–50.
11. Leknius C, Geissberger M. The effect of magnification on the performance of fixed prosthodontic procedures. J Calif Dent Assoc 1995;23:66–70.
12. Mamoun JS. A rationale for the use of high-powered magnification or microscopes in general dentistry. Gen Dent 2009;57:18–96.
13. Tibbetts LS, Shanelec D. Periodontal microsurgery. Dent Clin North Am 1998;42:339–359.
14. Koch K. The microscope: Its effect on your practice. Dent Clin North Am 1997;41:619–626.
15. Cuomo G. Posture-directed vs. image-directed dentistry: Ergonomic and economic advantages through dental microscope use. June 2006. Distributed by Sullivan-Schein. https://www.scribd.com/document/29204758/Continuing-Education-Posture-Directed-vs-Image-Directed-Dentistry-Ergonomic-and-Economic-Advantages-Through-Dental-Microscope-Use-June-2006. Accessed 21 July 2022.
16. Spear F. One clinician's journey through the use of magnification in dentistry. Adv Esthet Interdiscip Dent 2006;2:30–32.
17. National Institute for Occupational Safety and Health. Assessing Occupational Safety and Health Training: A Literature Review. DHHS (NIOSH) Publication Number 98-145. https://www.cdc.gov/niosh/docs/98-145/default.html. Accessed 8 June 2021.
18. Friedman M, Mora AF, Schmidt R. Microscope-assisted precision dentistry. Compend Contin Educ Dent 1999;20:723–737.
19. Murgel CA. Microscopio operativo para el odontólogo general: Una panacea o una solución definitiva para la clínica odontológica y la educación. Canal Abierto 2009;7:2–3.
20. Kinomoto Y, Takeshige F, Hayashi M, Ebisu S. Optimal positioning for a dental operating microscope during nonsurgical endodontics. J Endod 2004;30:860–862.
21. Valachi B, Valachi K. Mechanisms leading to musculoskeletal disorders in dentistry. J Am Dent Assoc 2003;134:1344–1350.
22. Parsell DE, Weber MD, Anderson BC, Cobb GW Jr. Evaluation of ergonomic dental stools through clinical simulation. Gen Dent 2000;48:440–444.
23. Ortiz Hugues JC, Adorno C, Ibarra-Mejía G. Estimation of moments in simulated dental cleaning task in four working positions. Presented at the 33rd Annual International Occupational Ergonomics and Safety Conference, 16–17 September 2021.
24. Blanc D, Farre P, Hamel O. Variability of musculoskeletal strain on dentists: An electromyographic and goniometric study. Int J Occup Saf Ergon 2014;20:295–307.
25. Valachi B. Ergonomic positioning: A few degrees add years to your career. Dent Today 2010;29:124–126.
26. Chaffin DB, Andersson GBJ, Martin BJ. Occupational Biomechanics, ed 4. Hoboken, NJ: John Wiley & Sons, 2006.
27. Zapara J. In focus: Microphotography using the dental operative microscope. Dental Town. https://www.dentaltown.com/magazine/article/5601/in-focus-microphotography-using-the-dental-operative-microscope. Accessed 5 April 2022.
28. Bud M, Jitaru S, Lucaciu O, et al. The advantages of the dental operative microscope in restorative dentistry. Med Pharm Rep 2021;94:22–27.
29. Erdmann WS. Center of mass of the human body helps in analysis of balance and movement. Appl Bionics Biomech 2018;2:144–148.

Index

Page numbers followed by "t" denote tables, "f" denote figures, and "b" denote boxes.

Index